THREE REALMS OF MANAGED CARE
SOCIETAL, INSTITUTIONAL, INDIVIDUAL

Resources for Group Reflection & Action

John W. Glaser
Ronald P. Hamel

Sheed & Ward
Kansas City

Sheed & Ward™ is a service of The National Catholic Reporter Publishing Company.

Library of Congress Cataloguing-in-Publication Data

Glaser, Jack.
     Three realms of managed care : societal, institutional, individual / John W. Glaser, Ronald P. Hamel.
        p.   cm.
     Includes bibliographical references (p.).
     ISBN: 1-55612-959-9 (alk. paper)
     1. Managed care plans (Medical care) I. Hamel, Ronald P., 1946-
II. Title.
RA413.G53   1997
362.1'04258--dc21

                                             97-33534
                                               CIP

Published by: Sheed & Ward
                  115 E. Armour Blvd.
                  P.O. Box 419492
                  Kansas City, MO 64141-6492

To order, call: (800) 333-7373

Cover design by Emil Antonucci.

This book is printed on recycled paper.

www.natcath.com/sheedward

Contents

III.

Readings in Individual Ethics of Managed Care

IV.

Processing Key Ideas and Processes for Reflection and Action

INTRODUCTION

WHAT THIS BOOK IS ABOUT

If you are planning for a year, plant rice;
for a decade, plant a tree;
for a century, educate.

Chinese Proverb

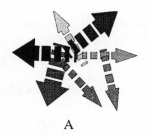

A

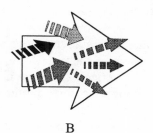

B

The two figures, A/B above, can help us understand what this book intends. Figure A represents the conflicting ideas, paradigms, emotions, motivations, interests, empowerments, assumptions, social forces, historical establishments, etc., that currently exist in our nation concerning health and health care. Figure B represents the kind of alignment in key ideas, paradigms, motivations, etc., that we need in order to have a reasonably just and effective health care system. (Despite the enormous contrast, there are solid reasons for hope: first, there are practical models operating in virtually every other developed nation of the West; and second, we have been able to move – at varying speed and with differing degrees of success – from the chaotic toward the consensual end of the continuum on other divisive issues: e.g., slavery, women's suffrage, ecology.)

Movement along this continuum, from chaos to growing consensus, will be slow and arduous – it will probably be measured in decades and generations rather than presidential terms. An essential dimension of this political, intellectual, cultural pilgrimage will involve individuals and groups in clarifying their understandings and evaluations. One key engine of this cultural evolution will be the thoughtful reflection of groups. This book intends to be fuel for this engine of sustained group reflection.

RESOURCES TO PROMOTE ETHICAL REFLECTION:

Health care is structured to provide direct service to acute need. This orientation has created a culture that is long on action and short on reflection. The present pace and direction of transformation in health care is exacerbating this situation. The same forces that are introducing new ethical ambiguities into health care are systematically and relentlessly wringing out of health care institutions the energy, time, and spirit needed to reflect on these broader and deeper ethical questions.

This book intends to resist this pressure to ever more frantic activity without reflection. It offers five things that offer a group some resources to resist this:

1) This book offers a clear ethical imperative that says: *don't just do something – stand there*. Stop what we are doing, step back from it and examine *what* we are doing, *how* we are doing it, *what impact* our actions and omissions are having on others, *who* are most impacted by our actions and omissions. Reflection on these and similar questions needs to be done with some consistency, not because what we are doing is bad but because it is complex, often unfamiliar, usually involving conflicting forces, without exception having hidden consequences – all of which can be overlooked in the press of doing our job. The more complex the issue, the more conflicting the forces, the more intense the pressures, the faster the pace – the more need to build in consistent structure for such ethical reflection. This ethical imperative suggests that a key measure of an organization's ethical quotient is the extent to which it has some solid infrastructure of reflection and self-examination; the extent to which it invests resources (especially the resource of senior management's time and energy) in examining some of the deeper issues from which our daily actions flow;

2) This book offers an *ethical paradigm* to organize our reflection on the complexity of managed care. It suggests that we think of three realms of ethical complexity: societal issues, institutional issues, and individual issues. This model will be discussed more in detail below and provides the framework for the structure of this book;

3) This book offers *articles for reflection and self-examination* on various aspects of managed care. These articles take specific issues – rationing, financial incentives, full disclosure – and develop their theme at some length to provide the basis for examination of the issue and its implications for the group conducting the discussion;

4) This books offers a *range of reflective processes* that a group can use to connect the content of these articles with the thinking and/or feeling of individuals in the group; with their institution's character and culture; with the systems and structures that shape the society in which we practice health care;

5) This book offers an imperative for action: "Don't just stand there – do something!" This book suggests that our reflection should lead to action – on all three levels – shaped by the more informed vision we have gained by our engagement with one another.

ETHICS AS INTERNAL, AFFECTIVE RESPONSE AND AS EXTERNAL EFFECTIVE ACTION FOR HUMAN DIGNITY

There is no single way to define ethics that trumps all other definitions. There are many solid ways to understand ethics. For our purposes it can help to think of ethics in terms of: *internal affective response for human dignity* and *external effective action for human dignity*.

THREE REALMS OF ETHICS*

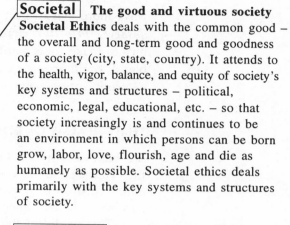

Societal The good and virtuous society
Societal Ethics deals with the common good – the overall and long-term good and goodness of a society (city, state, country). It attends to the health, vigor, balance, and equity of society's key systems and structures – political, economic, legal, educational, etc. – so that society increasingly is and continues to be an environment in which persons can be born grow, labor, love, flourish, age and die as humanely as possible. Societal ethics deals primarily with the key systems and structures of society.

Institutional The good and virtuous institution
Institutional ethics deals with the overall and long-term good and goodness of institutions (families, agencies, corporations). It attends to the health, vigor, balance, and equity of the institution's key systems and structures so that the institution can accomplish its mission while attending to its rights and duties vis-á-vis the individuals who make it up and the larger society in which it exists. Institutional ethics deals primarily with the key systems and structures of institutions.

Individual The good and virtuous individual
Individual ethics deals with the good and goodness of individuals. It attends to the balance and right relationships among various dimensions of a single individual (spiritual, mental, physical, emotional, etc.) as well as the rights and duties that exist between separate individuals. Individual ethics tends to deal with the behaviors and virtues of individuals.

Three Realms of Ethics, John W. Glaser, Sheed & Ward, Kansas City, MO

Center for Healthcare Ethics 440 South Batavia, Orange, CA 92668 (714) 997-7690

Internal affective response to human dignity: The starting point for ethics is our common experience that human persons and their world are precious – they deserve our reverence, esteem, and careful attention. This respect for human dignity is an inner, spiritual experience of awe, affirmation, good will toward human goodness; it has a boundless quality that wishes well to human persons and their world everywhere they exist. Ethics can be seen as those efforts that nurture, enable, celebrate, and deepen this inner affective sensitivity and response to human value and dignity.

External effective action for human dignity: When our *reverence* turns to *action – as it must to be fully human –* we face the human condition of hard choices. Since there is always more good to be done than we can do, and always more evil to be avoided than we can avoid, we must decide: *which good deserves priority?* Here, ethics serves human dignity by enabling the community to make these hard choices as humanely, consistently, effectively as possible. *A key function of ethics is to provide tools of discourse, discernment, and decision to the community of concern.*

THREE REALMS OF ETHICS

We believe that one key tool for making these hard choices is the paradigm that views ethics in terms of three distinct but interconnected realms: societal ethics, institutional ethics, and individual ethics (see, John W. Glaser, *Three Realms of Ethics,* Sheed and Ward, 1994).

This model of the three realms starts from the simple observation that human persons are *social individuals*. Both elements are essential: first, *we are unique, irreplaceable individuals*; second, our *individuality began and can only survive and flourish in social interdependence*. We can further make a rough distinction between two levels of social complexity: the larger civic community (nation, state, region) and smaller mediating social realities of family, business, church, etc. This thought model of individuals existing within larger social organizations – family, church, business – which in turn exist within a unifying social entity (state, nation) provides a helpful model for negotiating the hard choices. Applied to the ethics of managed care, this paradigm suggests that we proceed by addressing three realms of managed care: ethics of society managing care; ethics of institutions managing care; ethics of individuals managing care.

Managed Care As Societal Ethics

Societal ethics of managed care asks how society must understand and manage health care, what systems and structures must it have in place to be a reasonable and just society and to have a reasonable and just health care system?

The answer to this question grows out of many other complex issues: What is the nature and what are the limits of health care? Is it a social good, like fire and police protection, a commercial good, like cars and toasters, or a mix of the two? To what extent should market dynamics be encouraged, tolerated, prohibited? What is the relationship between health and human fulfill-

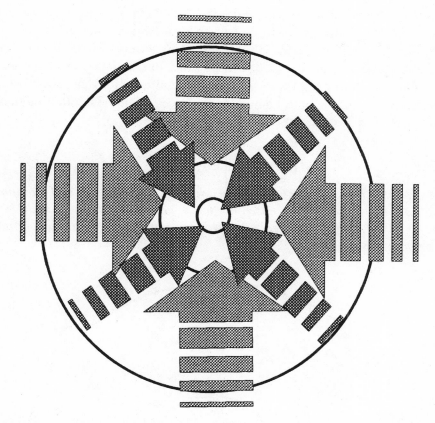

ment? between health and access to the other basic goods of our society and culture? between the other basic goods of our society and health status? What proportion of our societal resources should be expended on health care relative to the other social goods required to promote the common good – i.e., what is the relative societal value of schools, hospitals, jobs, safe streets?

Such issues are seldom given even short shrift in the current discussion of managed care. They are seen as different questions – public policy, health care reform. We believe that they are precisely questions of managed care on the societal level and need to be identified in their essential relationship to the other realms of managed care – institutional and individual. How we manage care on the societal level gives shape and sets limits to how institutions and individuals can and will manage care. The rationality or irrationality, the justice or injustice of managing care on this societal level cascades down into the smaller realms of institution and individual.

A brief example can make this connection clear. Treating health care as a market commodity (through key social mechanisms of tax structure, law, regulations, financing, etc.) on the societal level means that the connection between health care *service* and *wealth* will be strengthened and the connection between health care *service* and *need* will be weakened. This has powerful influence on the behavior of institutions and individuals, since both health care institutions and doctors will be financially punished for responding to health needs that are not tied to wealth. Societal systems and structures will punish those who serve the poor because of a prior societal determination that health care will be treated as a market commodity. The power of the societal realm to determine the ethical parameters of the lower realms – institutional and individual – is one reason that this realm is so important. Add to this the enormous complexity of these societal questions and we have ample reason to invest substantial community resources in the resolution of these societal issues in managed care.

MANAGED CARE AS INSTITUTIONAL ETHICS:

Institutional ethics of managed care addresses this broad and fundamental question: what elements are essential for a good and virtuous MCO? where does our MCO stand measured against these norms? how do we continuously improve our ethical status?

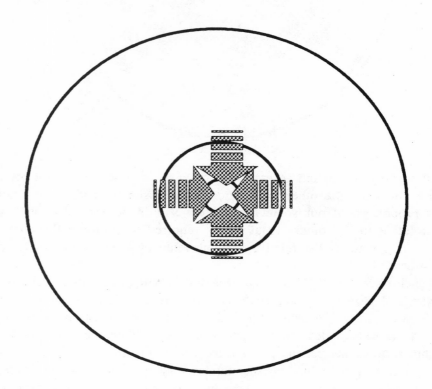

As we noted above, many of the systems and structures of an MCO are already predetermined by the systems and structures of the societal level. This means that there are severe limits to how much an institution can improve its own ethical quality without changing the societal systems that set the rules for its success and survival. This is the basis for an institutional ethical responsibility to educate the public and to engage in societal advocacy as important ways to change the societal parameters.

An ethically strong MCO should have explicit consensus about commitment to and effective systems and structures to realize priorities, such as the following (for a more inclusive list, see pp 139-40):

- personal, long-term relationship between primary care provider and patients,
- commitment to health promotion,
- shared understandings among all key publics about the nature, purpose and key mechanisms of managed care,
- clear statements of rights and responsibilities for members, providers and the plan,
- recognition that cost containment as an essential of quality care,
- culture of collaborative relationships and trust between primary care providers and specialists,
- financial incentives that include all concerned publics including patients,
- help for employers to understand dimensions of managed care beyond price,
- financial incentives spread over large groups,
- marketing that does not hide essential elements of managed care,
- strong presence of physicians at key points: e.g., governance, guidelines development, allocation decisions, appeals,
- systems and structures for continuous learning,
- commitment to advocacy for improving the societal parameters of health care policy.

Just as societal systems and structures set limits to options for institutions and individuals, so do the determinations and allocations of institutions set limits on the behaviors of individuals. Institutional ethics in managed care deserves a great deal of attention because: 1) institutions in their systems and structures have enormous and perduring impact on individuals – both those who staff such institutions and those who need access to these institutions to receive care; 2) institutional systems and structures are difficult to analyze and still more difficult to change.

MANAGED CARE AS INDIVIDUAL ETHICS:

Individual ethics of managed care involves the examination of the responsibilities and rights of individuals concerning themselves, other individuals and the institutions and societies within which they live.

For example, concerning health care professionals in a managed care setting, individual ethics would clarify their duties and rights vis-á-vis themselves, their patients (their own patients and the whole population of MCO patients), their health care colleagues, the MCO (concerning quality of care and participation in key functions shaping MCO infrastructure) and society (education of the public, advocacy for just health care policy and systems). Similarly, with other populations, individual ethics would aim at clarifying and promoting the actualization of what it means in a managed care setting to be a good and virtuous nurse, patient, therapist, case manager, marketer, administrator, receptionist.

NECESSITY OF ALL THREE REALMS

The ethics of managed care necessarily includes all three of these realms. We need to recognize that these are distinct arenas of responsibility and deliberation – *the forums, tools, methodologies and timelines vary greatly as we move from one realm to another*. If we overlook this fact, we will inevitably make serious mistakes. For example, we could mistakenly assume that ethical principles, for example, autonomy, have the same importance in the institutional and/or societal realm as they do in the individual realm. Or we could mistakenly think that conclusions which we legitimately draw on the individual level have direct and immediate implications on the societal level.

But we also *need to recognize the interrelationships, priorities, and interdependencies that exist between the three realms* – or we will make mistakes, such as thinking that we can remedy significant deficits on the societal level by compensating behavior of individuals or institutions. Or we might miss how powerfully societal injustices cascade down to severely limit the behavior of institutions and individuals.

By taking explicit and careful notice of all three realms of ethics – in their differences and their interdependencies – we have a better chance of respecting human dignity in all of its complex dimensions.

But when we pause and recognize that these are not merely realms of ideas and intellectual debate, but represent continents of emotion, personal self-definition, political and economic establishment, patterns of addiction and pathology (individual and national), we see why the road ahead is steep and tortuous, the burden unwieldy and weighty, the distance to be traveled far beyond the horizon. Facing such a formidable future, this book intends to be an expression of hope and a modest help for moving toward more just and reasonable possibilities.

PART 1

READINGS IN SOCIETAL
ETHICS OF MANAGED CARE

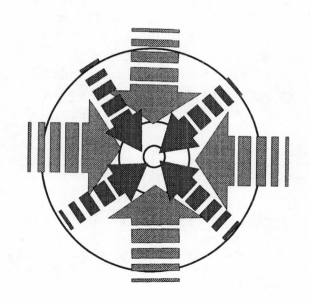

The articles in this section help us think about some select questions concerning how we as a society should understand and manage health care in order to have a reasonable and just society and a reasonable and just health care system. This engages us in two main sets of questions: 1) what are the meaning, the limits, and the role of health care relative to the other social goods that constitute the common good? 2) how should we allocate the limited resources within the health care good to reasonably and justly serve the countless needs for care?

The systems and structures that flow from our societal answers (or our failure to give answers) to such questions will, to a great extent, predetermine the possibilities for managing care on the institutional and individual level. Because of this cascading impact on the institutional and individual, because of the great depth and complexity of these issues, because of our wide divergence of interests, and because of our wretched track record as a society in explicitly addressing such issues, we cannot begin soon enough to dig into these questions

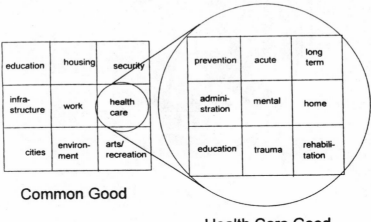

Common Good

Health Care Good

CHAPTER 1

SYMBOLS, RATIONALITY, AND JUSTICE: RATIONING HEALTH CARE

*Daniel Callahan**

PROPOSALS TO RATION HEALTH CARE IN THE UNITED STATES MEET A NUMBER of objections, symbolic and literal. Nonetheless, an acceptance of the idea of rationing is a necessary first step toward universal health insurance. It must be understood that universal health care requires an acceptance of rationing, and that such an acceptance must precede enactment of a program if it is to be economically sound and politically feasible. Commentators have argued that reform of the health care system should come before any effort to ration. On the contrary, rationing and reform cannot be separated. The former is the key to the latter, just as rationing is the key to universal health insurance.

One of the most important domestic tasks before the United States is to put in place a just and universal health care plan. Most people seem to believe, however, that such a plan would obviate the need for rationing health care, indeed that it is an alternative to rationing. This article argues that universal health care is neither feasible nor plausible without health care rationing. This contention is based not on some theory of just health care but on the experience of other countries that have some form of universal health insurance already in place. Each provides a decent level of health care. None provide all the health care that people might want, nor necessarily provide it in the way in which they would most like to have it.[1]

Why do these countries set such limits? Because early on they came to recognize what might be called the economic iron law of universal health care plans: to be affordable, they must be limited. If you want universal coverage, then be prepared to ration. If you are not prepared to ration, abandon all hopes of an affordable plan of universal coverage. To these general propositions, good for all countries and times, must be added a specifically American point: if we ever hope to persuade American politicians to enact a plan of universal coverage, then we must show them in advance how such a plan will control costs and how it will have built into it the ingredients to keep it from breaking the bank.

It is hard to say such things in the United States. Any discussion of the possibility of rationing health care in this country begins under a cloud. Symbolically, the very idea seems to offend a nicely tinted picture of ourselves as a rich, powerful nation, one that can afford to do whatever it takes to do whatever we want.[2] A nation that can put a man on the moon, that can afford Desert Storm and that can afford the S & L bailout is a nation that does not have to stint on health care. Especially for liberals, for whom the idea of universal health care has long been a high goal, any embrace of rationing seems a great betrayal. Since the main motive of the push for national health insurance has been coverage for the poor, the prospect of rationing care for that same group seems particularly offensive. It would seem to build into a program for the poor precisely those features that have so long burdened them: limits on what they can receive, while the more affluent can buy whatever care they want. As a symbol, then, rationing has nothing at all going for it. It seems, in fact, the perfect negative symbol of a weak and unjust society.

A strong and generous society must, however, be realistic if it is to do what needs doing. In case anyone addicted to symbols has not noticed, we have yet to enact universal health insurance in this country, and that failure comes at the end of at least 40 years of trying. It is at best naive, at worst obstructionist to continue invoking some idealized picture of ourselves to justify a failure to do what can be done, in a way it can be done, and to put in place something better than we now have. We can have universal health care in this country, but only if we can convince legislators and the American public that it is sensible and affordable. The only way to make such a case is to build an acceptance of rationing into it. What is now a negative symbol must be turned into one that is powerful and forthright: we can get what we need if we are prepared, in the process, to restrain ourselves. Rationing should be understood as a symbol of reasoning and restraint.[3] So understood, it can have great power, showing that we are concerned enough about the poor to pursue reasonable policies. However wonderfully symbolic, an anti-rationing policy is not reasonable.

There are other, more literal objections to rationing. It has often been taken for granted that health care rationing would positively harm the poor,[4] and that it would also represent a precipitate abandonment of efforts to control costs and eliminate waste.[5] It need not do any of those things. On the contrary, rationing is likely the only way in which we can improve care for the poor and manage our health care system in a more efficient manner. This article's argument, therefore, is strong and direct. Both as a symbol and as a way of organizing the health care system, rationing represents the most promising route available to us. Or, put somewhat differently, so long as it builds a method of rationing into it, the United States can have, and can afford a solid, decent and just health care system.

In this article, "rationing" means an action undertaken when there is: (a) a recognition that resources are limited, and (b) when faced with scarcity, a method that must be devised to allocate fairly and reasonably those resources. Rationing is the effort to distribute equitably scarce resources. This definition is consistent with much common usage.[6]

Rationing may be understood in a hard and a soft sense. The hard sense is that of the lifeboat at sea, where a limited amount of fresh water must be shared. In that case a method of distribution must be devised that accepts the fact that there will be no more water. The limits are absolute.

The soft sense of rationing is the kind that we confront with health care, and just about everything else, in the United States. The limits to resources are not absolute. We could, if we chose to do so, spend far more on health care. We could go from 12% of our GNP[7] to 20%. We could, for that matter, declare superb health care to be the main goal of American society, and the delivery of health care our main industry.

That is not likely to happen, and for a good reason. There are practical political constraints on how much money can be spent on health care. Limits are imposed by an unwillingness to pay higher taxes, to increase the burden of employers to provide health care, or to pay personally out of our own pockets. Public opinion polls time and again show that Americans, however high their aspirations for good health care, are not willing to pay an unlimited amount to have it or to put up with the restrictions that it might entail.[8] There are, as politicians know all too well, limits to a public willingness to tolerate tax increases, both across-the-board and for health care. For their part, employers cannot afford to jeopardize the overall fiscal soundness of their businesses by readily tolerating constant cost escalations. The Hastings Center[9] has had to put up with average increases of 25% per year for the past three years, and that is not atypical. Neither the Hastings Center nor more affluent organizations can afford to continue that pattern.

Limits are further imposed by common sense. We ought not to spend excessively on health care. We do so spend only at the cost of other important recipients of limited resources. We need a good educational system, good parks and roads, good welfare and poverty programs, good industrial research and development policies. Health is not the only human good. Despite the great hand-wringing about the state of our health care system, for the most part American citizens already have a high and adequate level of general health. No special national gain adheres in increasing average life expectancy, or in striving to conquer each and every human disease. It would be nice but it is not an imperative goal for the overall well-being of the country. Only a nation that overvalues health could think we need more of it.

This article speaks primarily about the health status of middle-class white people, those who can expect, on average, to live a long life, well into old age. But what is true of this group is not true of everyone. The most immediate pressing problem is whether we can bring to the poor and deprived the same benefits now available to the rest of us.

This article proposes the following ideal for the American health care system: every American should be guaranteed a decently adequate, affordable level of health care. The poor, in particular, should be provided such care. The goal would be universal access to decent care. The achievement of that goal will require significant government expenditures; the government should provide the base guarantee for the poor. Beyond that, a combination of employer and personal contributions can provide the remainder of the needed money for everyone else.[10]

Such a system would not make economic sense without some form of rationing, at least in its public government programs and its private employer programs. Why rationing? Because the government would be foolish to promise an unlimited system of health care, one devised independently of the costs of that system. No country on earth, including one with the most generous system, has done that. The government cannot say, in effect, that it will pay whatever it costs to give you the most advanced health care. It cannot promise to pay for every technological advance, however efficacious and however expensive. It cannot promise to help all of us live as long as we choose, regardless of what private hopes we might have. It cannot promise to jeopardize other important societal needs in the pursuit of improved health. It cannot promise to conduct an unending struggle against mortality.

The American Congress has a long memory. It can recall how it was assured, in 1972, that the kidney dialysis program would cost no more than $250 million per year in its fourth year of operation or thereafter.[11] It now costs over $3 billion per year.[12] Congress can recall when it put Medicare in place in 1965,[13] assured that the costs would be manageable. Those costs now are expected to bankrupt the Medicare Trust Fund within the next decade.[14] In neither case were any methods conceived or developed to keep the costs under control; they were not thought to be needed. With memories of this kind, Congress cannot be expected to initiate major new entitlement programs that do not show, in advance, how the costs are to be managed. Blank checks will not be issued. The estimate of the Pepper Commission in 1990, the major bipartisan congressional effort to formulate a response to the problem of indigent and long-term care, was a cost of an additional $69.6 billion per year for decent coverage.[15] That estimate was for the first year. Nothing was said about the second year; the Commission knew better than to do that.

In short, both because no nation on earth, not even the United States, can promise unbounded health care regardless of the cost, and because Congress will not pay for such health care, some system of limits must be put in place. I call such a system "rationing." It is rationing in the worst sense if it is capricious and discriminatory, as is our present method of using ability-to-pay as a way of limiting costs. But it can be rationing in the best sense of the term if, in response to the need for limits, a fair and reasonable way is developed to set and maintain these limits.

But of course, for symbolic and practical reasons, every possible rationale, every conceivable evasion, is being developed to avoid the need for rationing. If we could just organize our present system better, it is said, we could have all the necessary health care we want.[16] If we could simply wring the waste, inefficiency and excess bureaucratic and malpractice costs out of the system, we would not even have to think about rationing.[17] The basis for this faith in efficiency is not groundless. We know that our administrative costs are high, approximately 20% of all costs (in comparison with approximately 10% in Canada).[18] We know that a huge amount of money is spent in response to malpractice problems and on our present system of tort compensation.[19] These costs are not incurred in other countries.[20] We know that we waste billions of dollars on untested or misused technologies.[21] We know that most other developed countries can show as good or better mortality and morbidity outcomes for considerably less money per capita,[22] and for a smaller percentage of their GNP.[23] It is not, in a word, hard to show that we could get much better value for the money that we do spend, and probably even could get as good or better an outcome for less money.

Nonetheless, we are profoundly mistaken in believing that we should not move to open and conscious rationing *until* we have wrung all of that waste out of the system. This is a version of what this article calls the "best of all possible worlds fallacy": if we could just organize ourselves more efficiently, we could have all the necessary and affordable health care we want.

Why am I skeptical, and why do I call that a fallacy? Mainly because I have heard the same refrain again and again, for well over a decade now. Yet during that time, and despite a variety of highly touted cost containment programs, nothing has worked to any substantial degree to control costs or to bring much greater efficiency into the system. We have tried DRGs,[24] managed care,[25] HMOs[26] and competition.[27] No attempt has had any striking success, although some evidence shows that Medicare cost increases are being controlled.[28] The most that we can say is that costs might have been higher without these alternative health care plans. Overall health care costs continue to increase at two to three times the rate of inflation in general, and have risen even more sharply over the past three years.[29] Why should we expect some great shift in the historical pattern? Why, if we have failed for years in controlling costs, should we expect a transformation – the equivalent of a religious conversion experience – of the national character and of the present system?

It is a fallacy to conclude that because there is room for great savings, which there is, it therefore follows that we will have, and can get those savings. On the contrary, one can conclude only that the surest prescription to maintain the unfair and costly status quo is to continue talking about all the money that we can save simply by eliminating waste, malpractice, excess, and the bureaucracy. This is a method that surely has worked well toward that end so far. Nothing changes, and there is no prospect of any immediate change.

Why? We do not know how to eliminate waste in behavioral practice (even if we do in economic theory). In fact, we make things all the harder to change by posing the elimination of waste as an alternative to rationing. On the contrary, we will eliminate waste only by rationing. Only if we understand that we must live within restraints, and take the steps consistent with that recognition, can we contain costs. To be undertaken seriously, cost containment must be understood as another form of rationing. Responsible cost containment means saying "no" to some things that physicians, patients and administrators want. Serious cost containment means establishing practice guidelines and making them stick. Serious cost containment means the setting of priorities.

The issue before us is not a matter of cost containment *or* rationing. Both are necessary. They should be thought of as two sides of the same coin, not as alternatives. The experience of the European countries should sober those who think cost containment will make unlimited beneficial care available. Those countries – which have already in place most of the reforms that are desired in the United States – are beginning to feel the strain.[30] They have managed to control costs, but at the price of limiting services and requiring long waiting times for many procedures.[31] With the same demographic forces at work in those countries as here (that is, with an aging population), with an increase in high technology medicine, and with rising patient demands, these countries will be forced, as will we, into even more rationing in the future. They are quietly beginning their own rationing discussion – and are immensely curious to see how ours progresses.

The main concern about rationing in the United States is that the burden will fall upon the poor.[32] That is a serious problem. How can it be avoided? The overriding requirement is that this country have national health insurance and, with it, an adequate baseline of care. Inevitably, this baseline will have to be set at a level lower than the richest people can set their baseline. Rich people can hire limousines to get to their medical treatment, and helicopters to take them from their resort villas to daily psychoanalysis. Rich Americans can fly to Switzerland to use experimental treatments not available here. Rich people can seek out the very best specialists in the country and use them, rather than their local doctors. No conceivable government program could offer benefits of this kind to everyone. No private employee benefit program could offer them either.

Why should that matter anyway? What does matter is not whether the rich do better than the poor, but how well the poor do. The crucial issue is whether the baseline of care for the poor is set high enough to eliminate the most serious disparities between rich and poor. It could not eliminate all of them. It would take a totalitarian state to keep the rich and powerful from the health care that they want. The communist countries of Eastern Europe, as well as the Soviet Union, had the pretense of a single-tier, egalitarian system. The reality was that powerful party members got care not available to others, and that ordinary citizens had to bribe their way through the system to get good care. A democratic society would not even attempt to impose a single-tier system. It would invite corruption and evasion. But a democratic society would try to make certain that the poor have decent health care.

Yet if decent care is not the same as maximal care, how can the former be determined? It will, by definition, be rationed care. A fair system of rationing will have to set some priorities. If not everything can be made available to everyone, what is comparatively more or less important? The Oregon initiative is of great national importance. Using a combination of technical and economic considerations, and tempering them with expressed public values, that state has set up a system of priorities.[33] The Oregon legislators determined that it is better to provide health care coverage to everyone falling below the federal poverty line than to eliminate some people altogether in order to give virtually unlimited care to those who qualify. To make the new system possible, Oregon plans to limit services by means of its priority list.[34] The plan will also mandate that small businesses provide health insurance or pay into a pool that would make that insurance available to all employed persons.[35] The long-term goal is a system of universal health care in Oregon.

As the Oregon planners recognized, any process of rationing health care will have to find a way to balance medical judgment, economic possibilities, and public values. Yet it took some years to gain that insight. When the Medicaid program was established by Congress in 1965 to provide health care for the poor,[36] it specified that the indigent were to receive care that was "medically necessary)."[37] Congress did not, unfortunately (but perhaps deliberately), specify what that term meant or what means would be appropriate to make such a determination. It may have presumed that a purely medical standard of medical necessity could be determined.

If that is what Congress believed, it was wrong. As the intervening years have demonstrated well, it has turned out to be impossible to specify a purely scientific standard of medical "need," the basic concept that lies behind the idea of that which is "medically necessary." The problem is that "need" admits of no precise definition, ranging as it does over mental and physical needs, life-saving and life-enhancing needs. It is a notion, moreover, that is subject to different interpretations, open to the changed possibilities provided by technological developments, and subject to different evaluative interpretations. Thus although "medically necessary" and meeting health care "needs" have about them the ring of objectivity, they turn out to be flexible and malleable concepts. They combine both a descriptive and a normative content. They are at once scientific and moral concepts. This was not so obvious in 1965.

As time has gone on, it has been possible to trace a steady enrichment of our understanding of the ingredients necessary to specify a decent minimum of adequate health care.[38] Such care must include, in some plausible way, first, some reference to medical need; it must be rooted in commonly accepted notions of what people characteristically look for in health care. Yet, for all the above-mentioned reasons, it cannot use such a standard exclusively. Inevitably, many questions about the extent of those needs and the various evaluations required to deal with the borderline cases[39] will arise. Second, therefore, a decent minimum of average health care must include judgments about the efficacy of treatments to meet those needs; that is, what works and what does not work? A consideration of efficacy will, however, force a third set of considerations – that of the relative costs and benefits of different treatments. What will it cost to provide different benefits, and is there a good return on the money spent?

Next a decision will have to be made. If not everything can be afforded, what treatments and benefits are relatively more or less important? At this point, it should be abundantly clear that this question and those that preceded it require a central political component to be properly answered. Because these questions address fact and value, and the weighing of costs and benefits, they transcend a technical level. The questions call for collective judgment, judgment of a kind that will combine both expert and lay opinion. Thus, the fourth consideration is that a political process will have to be devised.

Since the political process almost certainly will encounter resource limitations, a question will then be raised: what is relatively more or less important in the provision of health care? The setting of priorities, then, will be a fifth consideration. How might that best be done? The state of Oregon has devised one method to do this,[40] and perhaps one could imagine others. Whatever other possible ways they might use to set priorities, however, other states would be wise in following the lead of Oregon in organizing community discussion of health care policy prior to the more formal political process of priority setting. Thus, the sixth consideration is the importance in giving the public not only a chance to express its opinions and preferences on priorities, but also a chance to become educated on the issues.

In a sharp attack on the Oregon approach to rationing and priority-setting, one of our most astute health care analysts, Lawrence D. Brown, wrote that "rationing has been elevated to the pantheon of fashionable solutions – competition, managed care, prudent purchasing, and more – that policymakers intermittently embrace as all-American answers to uncontrollable health care costs."[41] He then goes on to say that:

> [v]iewed in cross-national context, Oregon's contribution is mainly to show that, at least today in the United States, rationing is not a profound but a spurious issue. . . . The United States should worry less about rationing and more about constructing a rational policy framework whose watchwords are budgeting, planning, regulation, and negotiation. If the polity has declined to make those hard choices, rationing cannot save it from itself. American policymakers have not earned the right to ration health care, and the very policies that would earn it would eliminate much of the need to exercise it.[42]

Dr. Brown is wrong. First, rationing has not been proposed as one more solution to be put alongside competition or managed care, but as as a strikingly different kind of proposal. The other approaches were all designed to control costs within the present system of health care, not to change the system altogether. For many, in fact, they were meant as ways of avoiding rationing, as rationing is a generically different kind of approach. Second, what Dr. Brown proposes is perfectly sensible, but it *also* is fashionable. For what has been more common of late than to call for "a rational policy framework," and the national health insurance that would embody it? It is the best solution, and even those of us who support rationing would prefer such a framework as our starting point in an ideal world. But Dr. Brown neglects to mention that there has been no national progress of any significance toward that goal. There has been neither the political will for such a framework nor, in the face of budget deficits, any serious, politically potent constituency for it.

Third, the real genius of the Oregon initiative is that it starts with a recognition of limits as the first step toward a comprehensive health care system.[43] Its organizers say that in the present American political climate, the best way to get to Dr. Brown's goal of "budget, planning, and negotiation" is to concede at the very outset that rationing is necessary, and that the setting of priorities is the most sensible way of effecting it.[44] It is striking that none of the major national universal health care plans that have been proposed make any serious provision for controlling their costs. The Oregon plan takes limitation as its *point of departure* and then works from there.[45]

In effect, the Oregon plan stands Dr. Brown's approach on its head. Dr. Brown says that "American policymakers have not earned the right to ration health care, and the very policies that would earn it would eliminate much of the need to exercise it."[46] The organizers of Oregon's plan, by contrast, say that only by a willingness to embrace rationing – the orderly, equitable allocation of scarce resources – can we make progress toward universal health care, not the other way around.[47] They also say, moreover, that it is high time we stop talking about how a better, more rational system would obviate the need for rationing.[48] No universal health care system could avoid some degree of rationing. In any case, we are still far from significant national reforms, and the need now is to find a good starting point. In the absence of the will, leadership and public support necessary for national health insurance, Oregon is actually taking some real steps in that direction. The other states and the federal government are just talking.

The animus against rationing in the United States, symbolically and literally, expresses in one sense some of our most admirable values. Those are our touching faith in the power of efficiency, our commitment to egalitarianism, and our reluctance officially to pick upon the poor to test our social schemes. Rationing is thought to offend all of those values, and thus is rejected.

We deceive ourselves. Serious efficiency would require the equivalent of rationing, and that is why we have not achieved it. Our egalitarianism is more rhetorical than it is real. We tolerate a radically inegalitarian health care system as a day-to-day affair, but then rail against anyone – in the name of perfection – who would accept some degree of inequality as the first step on the way to a genuinely fair system. Although we carry out social experiments with the poor all of the time, including the crazy mess that is our Medicaid system, we rail at efforts to bring some sensible priorities and planning into that system, as Oregon is trying to do.

The usual approach to American problems is to say that since we are such a powerful and rich nation, we can afford nothing less than the best: the most lavish health care system and, with reform, the fairest and most efficient as well. So we reject any notion of limits, boundaries or self-restrictions. We live with our dreams. We should give them up and put realism and sobriety in their place. An acceptance of rationing would be a good place to begin. In fact, if we want national health insurance, it is likely to be the only feasible place to begin.

KEY IDEAS OF THIS ARTICLE:

- There is an iron law of universal access to health care: if you want universal health care coverage, then be prepared to ration; if you are not prepared to ration, abandon all hopes of an affordable plan of universal coverage.

- Rationing should be understood as a symbol of reasoning and restraint: we can get what we need if we are prepared, in the process, to restrain ourselves.

- "Rationing" means an action undertaken when there is: 1) a recognition that resources are limited, and b) when faced with scarcity, a method that must be devised to allocate fairly and reasonably those resources.

- "Both because no nation on earth, not even the United States, can promise unbounded health care regardless of the cost, and because Congress will not pay for such health care, some system of limits must be put in place. I call such a system 'rationing.' "

- We are profoundly mistaken in believing that we should not move to open and conscious rationing *until* we have wrung all waste out of the system.

- "We will eliminate waste only by rationing. Only if we understand that we must live within restraints, and take the steps consistent with that recognition, can we contain costs."

- What matters is not whether the rich do better than the poor, but how well the poor do. The crucial issue is whether the baseline of care for the poor is set high enough to eliminate the most serious disparities between rich and poor.

- A decent minimum of universal care will require explicit societal priorities.

- Some key ingredients necessary to specify priorities for providing a decent minimum of adequate health care include:
  - we must identify key health needs to be met;
  - we must identify treatments that are more/less effective in meeting these needs;
  - we must recognize that social priorities are a mixture of fact and value;
  - we must identify political processes that are effective in addressing the fact/value dimensions of these social priorities;
  - we must educate the community so that they are knowledgeable about the issues they are deciding;
  - we must organize and engage the community in processes of setting the priorities necessary for such fair rationing.

- Oregon offers us a good example of proceeding with such a process of rationing.

- The real genius of the Oregon plan is that it takes limitation as its *point of departure* and then works from there.

- The usual approach to American problems is to say that since we are such a powerful and rich nation, we can afford nothing less than the best; so we reject any notion of limits, boundaries or self-restrictions.

- In place of such an unrealistic dream, we should start with realism and sobriety – we should face the need to ration health care and make this the starting point of health care reform.

A SUGGESTED PROCESS FOR REFLECTING ON THIS ARTICLE:

(See pages 234-254 for other processes that might better fit your specific goals and objectives.)

1. There is an iron law of universal access to health care: if you want universal health care coverage, then be prepared to ration; if you are not prepared to ration, abandon all hopes of an affordable plan of universal coverage.
   ❏ strongly agree ❏ agree ❏ ? ❏ disagree ❏ strongly disagree

2. Rationing should be understood as a symbol of reasoning and restraint: we can get what we need if we are prepared, in the process, to restrain ourselves.
   ❏ strongly agree ❏ agree ❏ ? ❏ disagree ❏ strongly disagree

3. "Rationing" means an action undertaken when there is: 1) a recognition that resources are limited, and 2) when faced with scarcity, a method that must be devised to allocate fairly and reasonably those resources.
   ❏ strongly agree ❏ agree ❏ ? ❏ disagree ❏ strongly disagree

4. "Both because no nation on earth, not even the United States, can promise unbounded health care regardless of the cost, and because Congress will not pay for such health care, some system of limits must be put in place. I call such a system 'rationing.' "
   ❏ strongly agree ❏ agree ❏ ? ❏ disagree ❏ strongly disagree

5. We are profoundly mistaken in believing that we should not move to open and conscious rationing *until* we have wrung all waste out of the system.
   ❏ strongly agree ❏ agree ❏ ? ❏ disagree ❏ strongly disagree

6. "We will eliminate waste only by rationing. Only if we understand that we must live within restraints, and take the steps consistent with that recognition, can we contain costs."
   ❏ strongly agree ❏ agree ❏ ? ❏ disagree ❏ strongly disagree

7. What matters is not whether the rich do better than the poor, but how well the poor do. The crucial issue is whether the baseline of care for the poor is set high enough to eliminate the most serious disparities between rich and poor.
   ❏ strongly agree ❏ agree ❏ ? ❏ disagree ❏ strongly disagree

8. A decent minimum of universal care will require explicit societal priorities.
   ❏ strongly agree ❏ agree ❏ ? ❏ disagree ❏ strongly disagree

9. Some key ingredients necessary to specify priorities for providing a decent minimum of adequate health care include:

   • we must identify key health needs to be met
     ❏ strongly agree ❏ agree ❏ ? ❏ disagree ❏ strongly disagree

   • we must identify treatments that are more/less effective in meeting these needs
     ❏ strongly agree ❏ agree ❏ ? ❏ disagree ❏ strongly disagree

   • we must recognize that social priorities are a mixture of fact and value
     ❏ strongly agree ❏ agree ❏ ? ❏ disagree ❏ strongly disagree

- we must identify political processes that are effective in addressing the fact/value dimensions of these social priorities
  ❐ strongly agree ❐ agree ❐ ? ❐ disagree ❐ strongly disagree
- we must educate the community so that they are knowledgeable about the issues they are deciding
  ❐ strongly agree ❐ agree ❐ ? ❐ disagree ❐ strongly disagree
- we must organize and engage the community in processes of setting the priorities necessary for such fair rationing
  ❐ strongly agree ❐ agree ❐ ? ❐ disagree ❐ strongly disagree

10. Oregon offers us a good example of proceeding with such a process of rationing.
   ❐ strongly agree ❐ agree ❐ ? ❐ disagree ❐ strongly disagree

11. The real genius of the Oregon plan is that it takes limitation as its *point of departure* and then works from there.
   ❐ strongly agree ❐ agree ❐ ? ❐ disagree ❐ strongly disagree

12. The usual approach to American problems is to say that since we are such a powerful and rich nation, we can afford nothing less than the best; so we reject any notion of limits, boundaries or self-restrictions.
   ❐ strongly agree ❐ agree ❐ ? ❐ disagree ❐ strongly disagree

13. In place of such an unrealistic dream, we should start with realism and sobriety – we should face the need to ration health care and make this the starting point of health care reform.
   ❐ strongly agree ❐ agree ❐ ? ❐ disagree ❐ strongly disagree

IN LIGHT OF OUR DISCUSSION:

- as (executive committee, ethics committee, etc.), what are some next steps that we should take?

- as (hospital, home health agency, etc.), what are some next steps that we should take?

- what systems and structures call for special attention in order to improve the situation?

ENDNOTES

* Director and Co-founder, The Hastings Center, Briarcliff Manor, New York: Ph.D. 1965, Harvard University.

1. See Mark Pauly et al., *A Plan for "Responsible National Health Insurance," Health Aff.* Spring 1991, at 5, 20-21 (comparing experiences of the United States, the United Kingdom and Canada).

2. *See, e.g.,* Robert J. Blendon, *The Public's View of the Future of Health Care,* 259 JAMA 3587 (1988): Cindy Jajich-Toth & Burns W. Roper, *Americans' Views on Health Care: A Study in Contradictions. Health Aff.,* Winter 1990, at 149.

3. *Cf.* David C. Hadorn. *Emerging Parallels in the American Health Care and Legal-Judicial Systems,* 18 AM J.L. & MED. 73, 85 ("The problem of rationing merely is another instance of the need to balance individual welfare and public good.")

4. *See, e.g.,* Joan Beck, *Oregon Health Plan Faces the Reality of Care Rationing,* CHI. TRIB., Mar. 2, 1992, at C15; Spencer Rich, *Advocates for the Poor Hit Oregon Health Plan: Governor* Vows to Prevent Inadequate *Care, Wash. Post,* Sept. 17, 1991, at A3.

5. *See, e.g.,* David Lauter & Edwin Chen, *Health Care For All: Three Plans Compete,* L.A. Times, Nov. 11, 1991, at A1.

6. *See,* Kai N. Lee, *Salmon, Science and the Law in the Columbia Basin,* 21 ENVTL. L. 745, 776-77 (1991) ("[In] rationing lifesaving medical care . . . societies must attempt to make allocations in ways that preserve the moral foundations of social collaboration."); Pascal Fletcher, *Feeding Family Food Basket is Frustrating Chore in Cuba,* REUTER LIBR. REP., Sept. 30, 1991, BC cycle ("The authorities say the rationing system is the only way to ensure a fair distribution of scarce resources.")

7. *See,* George J. Annas et al., *American Health Law* 121 (1990) (11.1% of GNP in 1987); Robert D. Ray, *Health Tax Credits? A Sickly Idea: Here's A Plan That Won't Do Anything to Make the System Work. Wash Post.* Jan 26, 1992, at C5 (13% of GNP in 1991).

8. Robert J. Blendon, *supra* note 2, at 3588-90; Cindy Jajich-Toth & Burns W. Roper, *supra* note 2, at 153.

9. Daniel Callahan, Director.

10. This article does not address the details of that kind of system.

11. 118 *Congressional Record,* 33,004 (daily ed. September 30, 1972) (statement of Senator Hartke in sponsoring the end-stage renal disease section of the Social Security Amendments of 1972).

12. *See,* George J. Annas *et al., supra* note 7, at 890.

13. Health Insurance for the Aged Act, Public Library no. 89-97, 79 Stat. 290 (1965) (codified as amended at 42 U.S.C.A. §§ 401-426 (West 1991)).

14. John Holahan & John L. Palmer, *Medicare's Fiscal Problems: An Imperative for Reform,* 13 *Journal of Health Policy & Literature,* 53, 77 (1988).

15. *The Pepper Commission: United States Bipartisan Committee on Comprehensive Health Care, 101st Congress, 2nd Session, A Call for Action* 17 (S. Print 1990).

16. *See, Administration Health Care Proposals: Hearings Before the House Ways and Means Committee,* 102d Congress, 2d Session (1992) (statement of Dr. Louis Sullivan, Secretary of Health and Human Services) ("Indeed, one of our principles is to increase the efficiencies in our system because of my belief that we already have enough dollars in the system, but we're not spending them wisely."), *reprinted in* Federal News Service, February 20, 1992.

17. *See,* Amitai Etzioni, *Health Care Rationing: A Critical Evaluation, Health Affairs,* Summer 1991, at 88-95.

18. Steffie Woolhandler & David U. Himmelstein, *The Deteriorating Administrative Efficiency of the U.S. Health Care System,* 324 *New England Journal of Medicine,* 1253, 1255 (1991).

19. *See,* Leonard S. Weiss, *Finding the Remedies for Ills in Health Care: They Don't Come Easy, but They Do Exist, Newsday,* March 5, 1992, at 97 (defensive medicine adds more than $18 billion to health care costs).

20. *Cf.* Frank A. Sloan & Randall R. Bobvjerg, in *Medical Malpractice: Crises, Response and Effects, Health Insurance Association of America, Research Bulletin* 43 (1989) ("Price rises for liability coverage and heightened fears of litigation with its many uninsured costs have surely affected the climate of American medical practice.")

21. *Institute of Medicine, Assessing Medical Technologies* 211-27 (1985).

22. *See* George J. Schieber & Jean-Pierre Poullier, *International Health Spending: Issues and Trends, Health Affairs,* Spring 1991, at 106, 114 exhibit 6.

23. *Id.* at 110 exhibit 2.

24. Diagnosis-related group, which is a Medicaid payment plan under which hospitals receive a lump sum payment on the basis of discharge diagnosis, without regard to actual treatment provided. *See* George J. Annas *et al., supra* note 7, at 15-16, 234-48.

25. Under a managed care system, the patient chooses, or is assigned to, a primary care provider who then controls the patient's access to hospitals and specialists. Under most plans, the provider's income decreases if the provider approves expensive specialists or hospital care. *Id.* at 784.

26. Under a health maintenance organization system the patient pays a fixed sum and the organization promises to provide a defined package of inpatient and outpatient services. Doctors may be paid as salaried employees or on a fee-for-service basis. *Id.* at 774-75.

27. *See* Daniel Callahan, *What Kind Of Life: The Limits Of Medical Progress* 76 (1990).

28. *Id.* at 76-77. *See also* Sandra Christenson, *Did 1980s Legislation Slow Medicare Spending,* HEALTH AFF., Summer 1991, at 135.

29. *See* Stuart M. Butler. "Coming to Terms on Health Care," *N.Y. Times,* October 18, 1991, at A10.

30. See "Yesterday's Mirage: Why Britain's NHS Needs Competition," *The Economist,* Apr. 28, 1984, at 26 [hereinafter *Yesterday's Mirage*]; see also Daniel Callahan, *supra* note 27, at 88-89.

31. *See Yesterday's Mirage, supra* note 30, at 26-30.

32. *See* George J. Annas *et al., supra* note 7, at 70-74, 104-06.

33. *See* Charles J. Dougherty, "Setting Health Care Priorities: Oregon's Next Steps," *Hastings Center Rep.,* May-June 1991, at special supp. 1-16; Sara Rosenbaum, "Mothers and Children Last: The Oregon Medicaid Experiment," 18 *Am. J.L. & Med.* 97 (1992).

34. Sara Rosenbaum, *supra note* 33, at 104.

35. Act effective July 1, 1989, ch. 836, 1989 *Or. Laws* 836 (codified as amended in scattered subsections of *Or. Rev. Stat.* § 414 (1989)).

36. Pub. L. No. 89-97, § 1901, 79 Stat. 343 (1965) (codified as amended at 42 U.S.C.A §§ 1396a-1396u (West 1992)).

37. *Id.*

38. Charles J. Dougherty, *supra* note 33, at special supp. 3-4. *See also* Daniel Callahan, "Medical Futility, Medical Necessity: The Problem Without A Name," *Hastings Center Rep.,* July-August 1991, at 30.

39. For example coronary artery bypass surgery for an elderly person, or resuscitation efforts with a very low birthweight baby.

40. *Or. Rev. Stat.* § 414.720 (1991).

41. Lawrence D. Brown, "The National Politics of Oregon's Rationing Plan," *Health Aff.* Summer 1991, at 46-47.

42. *Id.* at 50.

43. *See* Daniel Callahan, "Ethics and Priority Setting in Oregon," *Health Aff.,* Summer 1991, at 78-87.

44. *See Oregon Medicaid Rationing Experiment: Hearings Before the SubComm. on Health and the Environment of the House Comm. on Energy and Commerce,* 102d Cong., 1st Sess. 19 (1991) [hereinafter *Hearings on Oregon Rationing*] (statement of Jean 1. Thorne, Director, Medical Assistance Programs, Dep't of Human Resources); *id* at 83 (testimony of Tina Castanares, Oregon Health Servs. Comm.).

45. *See id.* at 65 (testimony of Rep. Les AuCoin) ("Oregon's health plan is a program of expansion, not of limits.").

46. Lawrence D. Brown, *supra* note 41, at 50.

47. *See, Hearings on Oregon Rationing, supra* note 44, at 157, 160 (statement of Sisters of Providence of Oregon).

48. *See, id.* at 151 (statement of Peter O. Kohler, M.D., President, Oregon Health Sciences University): *id.* at 157 (statement of Sisters of Providence of Oregon).

CHAPTER 2

PRINCIPLES FOR MAKING DIFFICULT DECISIONS IN DIFFICULT TIMES

David M. Eddy

IN A PREVIOUS ARTICLE I DESCRIBED SEVERAL ISSUES OR "BATTLES" THAT will be particularly contentious in the coming decade.[1] They relate to the evidence needed to justify use of a treatment, to the need to balance a treatment's benefits against its costs, and to the autonomy of physicians to answer these questions for themselves. (I will use the word "treatment" very broadly to encompass any type of health intervention.) One way or another, these issues will be resolved in the next few years. Setting aside for a moment the actual solutions that are developed, the process by which these issues are addressed will provide one of the most visible displays of how the medical profession manages itself and responds to an urgent social need.

The main battlefield on which these issues will be resolved will be debates over coverage and guidelines for individual treatments. These debates will occur in every organization that is responsible for providing health care to a population – ranging from individual health plans to state Medicaid and public health programs to Medicare. The debates will occur over each new treatment as it is introduced, as well as over scores of old treatments that have been taken for granted for decades. The debates themselves will be unavoidable. The question is not whether they will occur, but how they will be conducted and the quality of the conclusions.

The key to ensuring that these debates will be resolved in an orderly fashion is to begin by agreeing on the principles that should guide them. If the principles are addressed in advance and in the abstract, the discussions can focus on the important medical, ethical, and economic issues. On the other hand, if there is no agreement on the principles at the beginning, each debate will quickly get mired in the details of the specific treatments and the narrow objectives of particular constituencies.

Ideally, there should be national agreement on a single set of principles. Whether health system reform will provide this type of leadership remains to be seen. However, the fact that no current proposal for national health system reform contains any such principles makes it unlikely that this will occur. In the absence of national leadership, every health care organization will need to create its own set of principles. To assist this process, this article proposes 11 principles that should guide debates over evidence and costs in organizations that must allocate shared or public resources to serve a defined population. "Shared" or "public' resources are accounts built from the contributions of many individuals – through such mechanisms as insurance premiums, health maintenance organization (HMO) dues, and state and federal taxes – to be spent on particular individuals who need treatments. If an individual is paying for a treatment by himself or herself, many of the principles, especially those dealing with costs, become moot.

When they are presented in the abstract, many of the principles will seem obvious, even trivial. However, applying them consistently will require some major shifts in our traditional ways of thinking and will have far-reaching consequences that will make many people uncomfortable. My hope is that health care organizations will debate each of the principles and either will agree with the ones I have proposed or will develop better ones. I also propose that, after it has reached agreement within itself, each organization should make its principles public. This should help achieve "informed consent" among providers, payers, consumers and patients, and should help all parties develop realistic expectations.

Despite their apparent simplicity, each of the principles begs questions about the best methods for implementing them. A full discussion of the methods is beyond the scope of this article. It is important to understand, however, that the validity of a principle does not depend on its ease of implementation. For two obvious examples, the principles "all men are created equal" or "turn the other cheek" are not invalidated by the difficulty of their implementation.

Finally, because the pressure of applying the principles will be most intense for the practitioners who actually provide the treatments, I will sometimes discuss the principles from their point of view. However, the applicability of the principles to all decision-makers should be apparent.

THE PRINCIPLES

The first principle deals with costs, because that is the main driving force behind the current changes in medical practice. It is really a premise.

1. The Financial Resources Available to Provide Health Care to a Population Are Limited.

It is crucial that every health care organization reach some conclusion on this premise, because all else follows from it. If this premise is false – if an organization truly faces no limits on the financial resources it has available for treatments – then the remaining principles become simple. In that case, it is acceptable for practitioners and patients to use any treatment they believe offers any hope of benefit. There is no need to determine that the treatment really does provide benefit (unless it also has harms), no need to consider its costs, and no need to make difficult trade-offs. The only remaining issues are to ensure that any harms of a treatment are out- weighed by its benefits and, if more than one treatment is available for a particular health problem, to determine which treatment offers the greatest net benefit.

Debates will be relatively peaceful because hardly anyone will be denied what they want.

The position that there are no limits on the amount of money that can be spent on health care treatments will be very popular. Not only do most of us have strong psychological, medical, and financial incentives to behave this way, but it is also a fact that until fairly recently there really were no practical limits on the amount of money available for health care. This is the traditional view, and it is the view that prevailed when most current treatments evolved into common use.

Unfortunately, there is strong empirical support for the premise that, whatever might have been true in the past, financial resources today are limited. Anyone working under capitation or prospective payment is obviously working under limits. Another impressive piece of evidence is the president's proposal for health system reform. It includes not only the limits imposed through the marketplace by competition, but an explicit, enforceable requirement that by 1999, the increase in a health plan's per capita premiums must be kept to the general rate of inflation. Even if this feature of the president's bill is eliminated in the congressional debates, its existence recognizes that the amount of money available for health care is limited. But the acid test for whether financial resources are limited is to simply ask those who are responsible for the budgets of health plans whether they have enough money to do everything everyone wants to do. If not, then the budget is limited.

If it is agreed that there are limits on the financial resources available to a health plan, there still might be disagreement over whether there are limits on the resources available for treatments. Some might feel that it should be possible for a health plan to respond to the financial limits by finding savings in administrative costs and hotel-type services, without having to impose any limits on the use of treatments. In another article, I will argue that it will not be possible to meet the limits imposed by the medical marketplace and health system reform through administrative efficiencies alone, and that the limits must affect the use of treatments. In the meantime, it is important to understand that the issue is not whether it should or should not be possible to meet the limits on resources without affecting the use of treatments. The critical question is whether the limits do affect the use of treatments. The presence of such things as precertification, utilization review, case management, fee schedules, restrictive formularies, and guidelines are all indications that the limits are affecting treatments. However, the acid test again is to ask those who are actually responsible for the budgets. Can they find all the savings they need from administrative efficiencies alone, or are they also looking at things such as drug utilization, use of expensive diagnostic tests, referrals to specialists, and expensive procedures? If they are, then the resources available for treatments are limited.

If it is agreed that the financial resources available to an organization for treatments are limited, or if an organization wants to prepare for the day when that will be the case, then it is important to examine the consequences of the first premise. Although there should be little debate about the next three items, because they follow directly from the limits on resources, it is important to state them explicitly.

2. Because Financial Resources Are Limited, When Deciding About the Appropriate Use of Treatment, It Is Both Valid and Important to Consider the Financial Costs of the Treatments.

3. Because Financial Resources Are Limited, It Is Necessary to Set Priorities.

4. A Consequence of Priority Setting Is That it Will Not Be Possible to Cover From Shared Resources Every Treatment That Might Have Some Benefit.

One does not have to think very hard to realize that these three principles raise the specter of rationing, which dictionaries define as the "distribution of scarce resources." This is obviously a very unpleasant idea to accept. But the only way to avoid it is to go back and reject the opening premise. Assuming that there is agreement on that premise, the next issue that arises is how the resources should be distributed and how priorities should be set. Most people will agree that the distribution should be equitable in some sense (although some advocacy groups for particular diseases or populations might prefer an unequal distribution in their direction). If we agree that the available resources should be distributed equally, the operational question is, how do we achieve that? This forces us to define the primary objective of health care.

5. The Objective of Health Care Is to Maximize the Health of the Population Served, Subject to the Available Resources.

This principle has enormous importance. In many ways, it is the fundamental principle that underlies the entire health care enterprise. On its face, it seems straightforward. However, as will become clear in a moment, it can be in conflict with another possible objective that we all cherish, which is to maximize the care we provide to every individual. Indeed, principle No. 5 goes to the heart of current debates about the individual vs. society.

To clarify this principle, we must first define what we mean by the terms "the population served" and the "health of the population." In the context of these principles, the population served is the total population for which the organization has a responsibility to provide care. In the current system, it is convenient to think of examples such as the members of an HMO or the people who qualify for a state Medicaid program. In the terms of health system reform, it is convenient to think of the population covered by a health plan. However, it is also important to recognize that providers can have a responsibility for people outside their particular organization — such as the uninsured who require emergency care.

Without trying to define precisely the outer boundaries of the population served, the important point is that it is much broader than the individual practitioner. It includes that practitioner's patients, plus the patients of all the other providers in the organization, plus all the well people for whom the health plan has responsibility.

Defining what is meant by the health of the population is more difficult and requires some concentration. However, it is important to work through the definition because it provides the foundation for resolving what is probably the most contentious issue we will face in the coming decade – setting priorities among treatments. The central point is easy to grasp: The health of the population is a "sum" of the health of all the individuals in the population. The justification for focusing on the sum across all the individuals is also easy to understand: if patients are going to be treated from a resource pool into which everyone in the population has contributed, then the distribution of resources from the pool should give equal and fair consideration to all the individuals who contributed. The more difficult concepts are how the benefits to an individual should be measured, and how the sum of benefits to a group of individuals should be calculated so as to maximize the total health of the population.

To help answer those questions and to distinguish principle No. 5 clearly from alternative principles that might be used to set priorities for treatments, I will pose a test question. This question requires that you think of a measure or scale that you can use to compare treatments. In this context the magnitude of a treatment's benefit should include both its benefits and harms (i.e., its "net" benefit), and should incorporate both the importance of the outcomes (e.g., survival from cancer vs. relief from a headache) and the probabilities that they will occur (e.g., a 50% vs a 2% increase in the cancer survival). Although there are formal scales that can be used for this purpose, you can think of a common-sense scale, such as a number from zero to 100, if you prefer. The scale should be cardinal in the sense that the score you assign to each treatment should reflect the relative magnitude of the benefit of that treatment compared with other treatments. Specifically, if you believe that the benefits of two treatments are such that one application of one treatment (i.e., to one patient) is equally desirable as two applications of another treatment (i.e., to two patients), you should assign the first treatment a score that is twice as high as the score you assign to the second treatment.

Some people – perhaps responding to a sense of egalitarianism – might object to the idea that treatments can be ranked in the manner I just described. To help think through this, you can ask yourself the following question. If you could choose to do only one of the following, which would you prefer to do: (1) prevent one 30-year-old mother of three from dying of cervical cancer, (2) treat a child who has noncyanotic tetralogy of Fallot (very debilitating, but not fatal), (3) repair a child's cleft lip, or (4) treat a person's tennis elbow? Unless you are truly indifferent about each of these four treatments, then a scale of benefits exists, and it is possible to rank treatments in order of their benefits. (If you are truly indifferent, then the principle for setting priorities should be to choose the least expensive treatment first. In this example, first priority would go to fixing all the tennis elbows, second priority would go to repairing all the cleft lips, and so forth.) A second possible objection is that even if it is possible to rank the benefits in their order of importance, you might not believe that it is possible to develop a cardinal ranking that implies a willingness to trade treatments across patients. To think about that, try the following – I am going to assume you assigned a higher benefit to treating a case of tetralogy of Fallot than to repairing one cleft lip. Now suppose you could either (1) treat one case of noncyanotic tetralogy of Fallot, or (2) repair 10 cleft lips, or 100 cleft lips, or every cleft lip there is in the world. If there is any number of cleft lip repairs that you would consider as desirable as treating one case of tetralogy of Fallot, then there is a measure of benefit that has the properties we want. Finally, you should not worry about whose values would be used to make choices like these. To help focus on the principles, you can assume that the country will use your values to score the treatments.

Now that we have clarified what we mean by the magnitude of benefit of a treatment, we can pose the test problem. To get right to the point, I am going to construct the problem so that it raises the most difficult and agonizing comparison. In reality, most decisions will be easier than this. Imagine that you have enough money to offer only one of the following two treatment programs. Program A provides 60 units of benefit to one person. Program B provides 30 units of benefit to five people (i.e., each of the five people gets 30 units of benefit, for a total of 150 units). Given these definitions (and remember that the benefits of the treatments are based on your values), principle No. 5 says that, if you can do only one of these programs, you should give higher priority to program B than to program A. The reason is clear: program B does more to increase the health of the population than does program A.

This is a head-on collision in the debate about the individual (the one patient who would receive treatment A) versus society (the five who will receive treatment B), and resolves the debate in favor of society. It is also consistent with the "the greatest good to the greatest number." Astute readers will read that if the values assigned for the benefit of each treatment have the property described, then there is no choice but to prefer program B. By assigning scores of 60 to treatment A and 30 to treatment B, you were expressing a willingness to trade one application of A for two applications of B. This test problem offered you an opportunity to trade one application of A for five applications of B, which would obviously be a desirable trade. Nevertheless, some might want program A because, on a patient-by-patient basis, it provides a greater benefit.

This principle will cause great discomfort to practitioners when one of their treatments receives a low priority. Because this discomfort will probably make this the most controversial principle, it is helpful to address it directly. We should begin by recognizing that the discomfort is caused by a noble instinct, which is to try to help any individual we see who is in trouble. We should also recognize that the instinct has many desirable qualities. The most obvious is that it helps ensure that the patients we see receive the best possible treatment. Having said this, however, it is also important to understand some of the drawbacks of the instinct and to contemplate some ways to alleviate the discomfort it causes.

The first point is that if we give in to the discomfort and follow our instincts, that will not solve the problem of how we should set priorities. That is, maximizing the care we provide to our personal patients is not really an alternative to principle No. 5. To the extent that it sets priorities at all, it sets priorities according to types of patients (e.g., "my patients" versus "someone else's patients"), not types of treatments. Such a position is obviously difficult to defend. But beyond that, trying to maximize the care we give to our personal patients is not a successful method for achieving the requirement that we keep costs within a limited budget. In terms of the test problem, if each practitioner seeks to maximize the treatments of his or her personal patients, practitioners with patients who need treatment A will order treatment A for their patients, and practitioners with patients who need treatment B will order that treatment for their patients. The end result is that both program A and program B will be done, which exceeds the specified limit. This is just what is happening in our current health care system; our attempts to maximize the care we give to our individual patients have led to increases in costs that are unacceptable (the opening premise). This is occurring even though a large portion of the population is omitted from this strategy altogether, because it has no coverage at all. So the first point is that giving in to our discomfort and seeking to maximize the care we provide to our personal patients not only fails to solve the problem of resource limits, it makes it worse.

A second point is that applying principle No. 5 will not mean that patients will be denied treatments that have high value. To address a more specific fear, a treatment will not receive a low priority simply because it is expensive. An expensive treatment would receive a low priority only if its benefits were too small to justify its cost.

A third point is that we have already been making these types of choices for decades. That is, despite our perceptions that we are maximizing the care we give to personal patients, we already make choices that fail to do that. Medicine is filled with indications, thresholds, and limits that are based on an implicit judgment that some amounts of benefit are just too small to be worth the cost. Frequencies of screening tests and indications for imaging tests are just a few examples. Although the choices will become more explicit and intense in the future, appreciation of this long tradition should help relieve some of the discomfort.

A fourth point is that at least some of the discomfort of withholding program A from one patient, even your patient, should be soothed by realizing that five other patients will receive treatment B, which we have agreed will provide greater total benefit. Conversely, if your patient receives treatment A, you will have to deal with the fact that five patients will be deprived of treatment B. A final approach for dealing with the discomfort is to ask yourself which health plan you would want your newborn grandchild to join: one that offers program A or one that offers program B.

If you decide not to accept the principle I have proposed for setting priorities across treatments, then you will need to agree on some other principle for setting priorities. We have seen that trying to maximize the care we give to our personal patients is not an alternative, because it sets priorities across people, not treatments, and because it does not achieve the required objective of keeping costs within the required limits. Some other ways that are sometimes used to set priorities include family and friends over strangers (e.g., physicians' spouses get special treatment); income and family status (as Medicaid now does); the prominence or visibility of an individual patient (e.g., a politician or patient covered in the nightly news); the squealing wheel (e.g., patients who threaten to sue); political correctness; the lobbying power of a particular advocacy group; the visibility of a disease (e.g., cancer); the technical appeal of a treatment (e.g., transplantation); and fear of malpractice. Although all these are real and can sometimes be justified in special circumstances, and although each will undoubtedly continue to play some role in individual decisions, it is clear that none of them is suitable as a general principle.

There are, however, two other candidates for a principle for setting priorities that might receive serious consideration. One is to give priority to treatments in the order of the severity of the health problems they treat. For example, this approach might give first priority to treatments that address urgent, life-threatening problems; next priority to treatments that address problems that are life-threatening but more chronic; third priority to treatments for problems that are severely debilitating but not life-threatening, and so forth. Although this approach has a strong surface appeal – apply the most resources to the most serious problems – it has some very questionable implications. For example, application of this strategy would provide all possible treatments for an acute life-threatening disease, no matter how futile the treatment, how low the probability of success, or how high the cost. Indeed, this principle does not even use information on the amount of benefit provided by different treatments. Rather, it is based on an assumption that if a treatment is used for an important problem, it must have an important benefit, which is clearly not always true. Here is a test question. If you could do only one, which would you prefer: treatment that increased the chance of surviving a heart attack from 92% to 92.5%, or a treatment that would completely restore all function to a 12-year-old quadriplegic? This approach would require that you choose the former because it addresses an acute life-threatening problem.

The other possible principle for setting priorities across treatments that might receive serious consideration is to rank treatments by the amount of benefit they provide to an individual patient. This is preferable to the one just mentioned, because it does at least consider the actual benefits of a treatment. However, because this approach ignores the cost of the treatment, it does not take into account the number of patients who could actually be helped, within the available budget. In terms of the test problem, this strategy would give priority to program A over program B, because treatment A provides 60 units of benefit per patient, whereas treatment B provides only 30 units of benefit per patient. However, this strategy would miss the fact that for the same amount of money, treatment B could be given to five times as many patients as could treatment A. If you want to take into account the costs of a treatment (which affects the number of patients it can be used to help), and if you want to be consistent with the way you have determined the benefit of a treatment, then you need to choose principle No. 5, which maximizes the total benefit a treatment can provide to the population.

Principle No. 5 has many implications. One that has already been alluded to should be made explicit.

6. The Priority a Treatment Should Receive Should Not Depend on Whether the Particular Individuals Who Would Receive the Treatment Are Our Personal Patients.

In terms of the previous example, we should give priority to program B over program A, even if the individual helped by program A is our own patient, while the five people helped by program B are not. This principle resolves part of the debate about the difference between "statistical" versus "identifiable" lives; it says that a statistical life (a person who is not your patient) is just as real and important as an identifiable life (a person who is your patient). We need this principle to avoid the obvious contradictions that would arise from the fact that lives that are "identifiable" to one practitioner are "statistical" to another practitioner and vice-versa. Those who disagree with this principle will have to justify a position that their patients are more important than the patients of their colleagues. They will also have to find some way to reconcile the conflicts that will constantly arise when their colleagues apply the same logic to shift resources back to their own patients.

This principle has important implications for the idea that the physician should serve as the advocate of his or her patients. It reminds us that in organizations that cover the costs of treatments from shared resources, physicians' responsibilities extend beyond their personal patients to affect all the patients in the population they help serve. When resources are limited, and when treatments are being paid for from a resource pool to which everyone contributed, a better maxim is that the physician should serve as an advocate of all the individuals in the population, not just their personal patients.

This principle also has implications for "rationing at the bedside." I interpret this term to mean requiring the practitioner to personally make a specific decision to withhold some beneficial treatment from a specific patient because of its cost. Principle No. 6 does imply that some beneficial treatments will be withheld from some patients, as has occurred in the past. However, there is nothing in this principle that forces the individual practitioner to make these decisions one-on-one at the bedside. A far better way to implement these decisions is to use the traditional approach of imbedding them in guidelines, which the physicians and patients can then follow without having to suffer the anguish of making the decision themselves. A current recommendation for annual mammograms is an example – compared with six-month examinations, it is rationing.

Before we leave this topic, it is useful to address the remaining part of the debate about statistical versus identifiable lives – the "rule of rescue."[2] The rule of rescue is based on the observation that many people place a very high value on attempts to rescue individual identifiable people who face a desperate problem, provided that they fit certain criteria. A prototypical example is a child who falls down a well. Flying a child from Bosnia to the United States for surgery is a recent example. The main criteria are that the circumstances should be extraordinary (e.g., relatively rare and very dire), that we can identify with the individual who is in distress, and that the incident has high symbolic value. For example, we do not apply the rule of rescue to a homeless man dying of pneumonia over a steam grate.

There is no denying the fact that the rule of rescue is real – both as individuals and as a society, we do feel a strong instinct to help particular individuals who attract our attention like that. Fortunately, this instinct can be accommodated in the fifth principle. The key is in the measure of benefit. Imagine that treatment A is a long-shot heroic attempt to save the life of a particular individual at a cost of $400,000. If we place such a high value on trying to rescue this individual that we are willing to allocate the $400,000 to this treatment, even if that would mean withholding more mundane but more effective treatments from a larger number of patients, we can accommodate that by assigning an extremely high score to the treatment, "long-shot heroic treatment of this particular individual." If we set the score of this treatment high enough, it will always receive priority, no matter how many resources it might pull from other treatments. The point here is not to make a judgment about the appropriateness of the rule of rescue, but to say that, to the extent that society wants to allocate resources to trying to rescue particular individuals, the fifth principle can accommodate that.

If the principles I have proposed thus far are accepted, then several additional principles follow from them.

7. Determining the Priority of a Treatment Will Require Estimating the Magnitudes of Its Benefits, Harms, and Costs.

Although this is not really arguable, because it follows directly from the fifth principal, it has very important implications. Specifically, it will require a shift in medical decision-making from qualitative thinking to quantitative thinking. Qualitative thinking looks only at the possibility of benefit. Representative phrases are that a treatment should be used if it "might be beneficial," if it provides "any hope of benefit," if it is "all we have to offer," or if it is "the patient's only hope." Elsewhere I have called this the "criterion of potential benefit."[3] In contrast, quantitative thinking requires that we do our best to determine that there actually is benefit, and that we estimate the magnitude of the benefit (the "criterion of actual benefit"). In terms of the test problem for principle No. 5, it is clear that we would have no basis for choosing between treatments A and B if all we could say about them is that they both have some benefit. To have any hope of allocating resources to the best treatments, we have to estimate the actual benefits of the treatments. The main objections to this principle will be the extra work involved to make the estimates and the prohibition of vague testimonials. However, seeking estimates of benefits, harms, and costs is clearly consistent with the time-honored concepts of intelligent decision-making and informed consent.

Applying this principle will mean that we will have to obtain the estimates of the benefits, harms, and costs from some source, which leads to principle No. 8.

8. To the Greatest Extent Possible, Estimates of Benefits, Harms, and Costs Should Be Based on Empirical Evidence. A Corollary Is That When Empirical Evidence Contradicts Subjective Judgments, Empirical Evidence Should Take Priority.

In the past, the most common method used to determine the values of different treatments has been to simply ask those who should know – to draw on clinical judgment, expert opinion, and professional consensus. Principle No. 8 says that we should first examine whatever actual evidence exists about the treatment and that we should use axiom-based methods to interpret that evidence. This principle obviously has important implications for the methods used to design guidelines.[4,5]

Although all the principles face methodological problems, applying this one will be especially difficult, which is why it begins with the qualifier, "to the greatest extent possible." Because the available evidence for a treatment is never perfect, it is rarely possible to rely entirely on empirical evidence, and some expert judgments will always be necessary. The intention of this principle is not to say that expert judgment will never play a role in evaluating a treatment. Rather, the intention is to ensure that there is a systematic search for evidence, that whatever evidence does exist is given priority, and that expert judgments are limited to specific "technical" questions for which medical expertise is required, rather than to global judgments about a treatment.

If there is agreement about the sources of information for making decisions about treatments, the next question is the actual criteria that a treatment must meet before it should be promoted. They are addressed in the next principle.

9. Before It Should Be Promoted for Use, a Treatment Should Satisfy Three Criteria.

- There should be convincing evidence that, compared with no treatment, the treatment is effective in improving health outcomes.

- Compared with no treatment, its beneficial effects on health outcomes should outweigh any negative effects on health outcomes.

- Compared with the next best alternative treatment, the treatment should represent a good use of resources in the sense that it satisfies principle No. 5.

This is really a summary of the preceding principles in the sense that if a treatment satisfies the others, it will automatically satisfy this, and vice-versa. Nonetheless, it is convenient to have this type of checklist to apply to specific treatments. This principle also highlights some important issues.

First, the principle addresses the "promotion" of a treatment. Examples of policies or activities that actively promote a treatment are initiation of coverage (if the treatment is not already covered), guidelines that recommend its use, inclusion in quality improvement criteria or quality "report cards" that encourage high rates of use, advertising or marketing that promotes use, malpractice sanctions for nonuse, and so forth. Thus, this principle is fairly lenient in that it does not stipulate that a treatment cannot be used unless it satisfies the criteria. For example, a treatment such as radical prostatectomy for prostate cancer that clearly has harms and costs, but that has not been documented to have benefit,[6] could still be used as an "option."[7] The principle says only that it should not be promoted through policies such as those just listed. An aggressive program to reduce waste and improve quality would have to tighten this principle to say that a treatment should be discouraged if it fails to satisfy the criteria.

Second, this principle works for treatments that are designed to be cost-saving, as well as for treatments that provide additional benefit at an additional cost. By the first and second criteria, a cost-saving treatment would still have to be effective and beneficial, and the third criterion would require that the amount of savings more than offsets any decrease in benefit, either by enabling the treatment of more patients with this health problem or by shifting resources to more cost-effective treatments for other health problems. Similarly, if a treatment increases benefit but at a higher cost, the third criterion requires that the increase in benefit from this treatment be large enough to make up for the loss of benefit caused by funneling resources from other treatments.

Third, the emphasis on health outcomes – outcomes that patients can experience and care about, such as life and death, pain, suffering, disability and appearance – is important. When the only available evidence addresses immediate outcomes (e.g., serum cholesterol, shrinkage of a tumor on roentgenogram, normalization of enzyme levels), the case for a treatment must include additional evidence that a change in intermediate outcomes caused by the treatment causes an improvement in health outcomes.

Fourth, the second criterion raises a new issue, which is the need to make comparisons between benefits and harms. The obvious question is this: who should make those judgments?

10. When Making Judgments About Benefits, Harms, and Costs, to the Greatest Extent Possible, the Judgments Should Reflect the Preferences of the Individuals Who Will Actually Receive the Treatments.

The justification of this principle is obvious: because it is patients who will actually live or die by the outcome, and who will eventually pay the costs, it is they who should have the primary say in what is done to them (including having nothing done). Application of this principle will vary, depending on the nature of the decision and the patient. The most obvious way to apply this principle is to present each patient, one by one, with information about the benefits, harms and costs of alternative treatments, and to let them choose. Unfortunately, this one-on-one approach is often not feasible, or is inappropriate because of other factors that are important to consider. For example, this approach would be unfeasible if there were time; if the options were too confusing for the patient, despite every effort by the physician to make them understandable; if the patient were unconscious or incompetent; or if the patient simply did not want to participate actively in the decision. This approach would also be inappropriate if the alternative treatments had different costs, because it is unrealistic to expect patients who do not actually pay the costs to incorporate the costs accurately in their decisions. However, the presence of these problems does not change the principle itself, which is that to the greatest extent possible, the preferences applied should be the preferences of those who will actually receive the treatment.

For many treatments, the quality of the evidence and the relative magnitudes of benefits, harms, and costs will make it easy to apply the ninth and 10th principles. However, for many other treatments there will be real debates about whether they are effective, beneficial, or a good use of resources. To resolve these debates, it is necessary to determine who should bear the burden of proof. This is addressed in the last principle.

11. When Determining Whether a Treatment Satisfies the Criteria of Principle No. 9, the Burden of Proof Should Be on Those Who Want to Promote the Use of the Treatment.

Whichever way the burden is placed – on those who want to use the treatment before there is convincing evidence of effectiveness and benefit, or on those who want to wait for better evidence – there will be some mistakes made. Placing the burden on proponents will retard the use of some treatments that, although we might not be able to demonstrate it yet, are actually effective, beneficial, and a good use of resources. Conversely, placing the burden on skeptics to prove that a treatment is ineffective or harmful will allow some treatments to slip through that are actually ineffective, a poor use of resources, or even harmful. Based on an analogy with our court system, a case might be made that a treatment should be considered "innocent" (e.g., effective, beneficial, cost-effective) until it is proven guilty. I have proposed the opposite, for the following reasons.

First, there are many precedents. Begin with the Hippocratic Oath, which admonishes us to "first, do no harm," and with the fact that harm takes many forms, including the morbidity and cost of a treatment. I interpret the oath to mean that before we do things to patients, we should have good reason to believe that they will be benefited. This principle is also consistent with the Food and Drug Act and its amendments, which require evidence of safety and efficacy before drugs can be marketed. It is also consistent with the scientific tradition of the last several centuries, in which ideas progress in an orderly fashion from hypothesis through testing to implementation, not from hypothesis directly to implementation.

Second, if proponents of a cost-increasing or harmful treatment did not have to establish its effectiveness, there would be virtually no brake on what could be promoted. For an absurd example, suppose someone wanted to promote the placement of patches of tar pitch behind the left ear as a treatment for thalassemia. Because there is no evidence at all about this treatment, opponents would not be able to prove that it was ineffective, and proponents would be free to promote its use.

Third, although errors will occur no matter who bears the burden of proof, the errors are much easier to reverse if the burden is on the proponent. If the use of a treatment is retarded because the evidence of benefit is not yet convincing, that problem can be corrected by doing the necessary research. For a truly effective treatment, the "cost" is a delay, not the permanent elimination of the treatment. On the other hand, if a treatment of unknown benefit can be promoted without requiring evidence of effectiveness, then there is no need to do the necessary research. In most cases the research will never be done (indeed, such research might well be labeled by proponents as unethical), and no one will ever know if the treatment is effective, beneficial, or a good use of resources. The difficulty of finding funding for research complicates the implementation of this principle. However, that problem must be solved by increasing the funds for research, not by changing the principle and opening the gates to all treatments anyone wants to promote.

A final reason to require evidence of effectiveness and benefit before promoting a treatment is that patients and practitioners need the information this principle would require in order to make intelligent decisions.

NEXT STEPS

These principles raise many questions. One of the most important is this: will it really be necessary to ration treatments? More specifically, even if it is agreed that financial resources are limited, will it be possible to achieve all the necessary savings from administrative and logistical efficiencies, without having to cut into the content of medical care? That will be the subject of the next article.

KEY IDEAS IN THE ARTICLE:

- Limited health care resources will increasingly require more and more decisions about how to allocate those resources.

- The most vexing questions this raises are what principles will guide such decisions and whence these principles should come.

- There should be a single set of principles to guide national debate and decision-making.

- In the absence of a single set of principles, however, each health care organization will have to create its own principles.

- As a first step, Eddy proposes 11 principles, which he hopes each health care organization will debate and either agree with or develop better ones.

- Once organizations reach agreement on these principles, they should be made public.

A SUGGESTED PROCESS FOR REFLECTING ON THIS ARTICLE:

(See pages 234-254 for other processes that might better fit your goals and objectives.)

Eddy's 11 principles are listed below. You are asked to indicate your level of agreement or disagreement and the reason(s) for your choice.

The first four principles consist in assumptions about allocation. Indicate your level of agreement with each principle. Identify areas of agreement and disagreement among members of the group. Discuss areas of disagreement, if there are any, and try to arrive at some consensus. Formulate that consensus in statements that would replace Eddy's.

1. The financial resources available to provide health care to a population are limited.
   ❏ strongly agree ❏ agree ❏ ? ❏ disagree ❏ strongly disagree
   Comment: _____
   _____

2. Because financial resources are limited, when deciding about the appropriate use of treatments, it is both valid and important to consider the financial costs of the treatment.
   ❏ strongly agree ❏ agree ❏ ? ❏ disagree ❏ strongly disagree
   Comment: _____
   _____

3. Because financial resources are limited, it is necessary to set priorities.
   ❏ strongly agree ❏ agree ❏ ? ❏ disagree ❏ strongly disagree
   Comment: _____
   _____

4. A consequence of priority setting is that it will not be possible to cover from shared resources every treatment that might have some benefit.
   ❏ strongly agree ❏ agree ❏ ? ❏ disagree ❏ strongly disagree
   Comment: _____
   _____

The next two principles begin to address how resources should be distributed and priorities set. Again, indicate your level of agreement with each of these principles. Identify areas of agreement and disagreement. Discuss areas of agreement in view of achieving some consensus. Formulate the consensus as a replacement principle.

5. The objective of health care is to maximize the health of the population served, subject to available resources.
   ❏ strongly agree ❏ agree ❏ ? ❏ disagree ❏ strongly disagree
   Comment: _____
   _____

6. The priority a treatment should receive should not depend on whether the particular individuals who would receive the treatment are our personal patients.
   ❑ strongly agree ❑ agree ❑ ? ❑ disagree ❑ strongly disagree
   Comment: _____

   _____

More specific principles follow from the above. They actually provide guidelines for making allocation decisions. Use the process described above to address the next three items.

7. Determining the priority of a treatment will require estimating the magnitude of its benefits, harms and costs.
   ❑ strongly agree ❑ agree ❑ ? ❑ disagree ❑ strongly disagree
   Comment: _____

   _____

8. To the greatest extent possible, estimates of benefits, harms, and costs should be based on empirical evidence. A corollary is that when empirical evidence contradicts subjective judgments, empirical evidence should take priority.
   ❑ strongly agree ❑ agree ❑ ? ❑ disagree ❑ strongly disagree
   Comment: _____

   _____

9. Before it should be promoted for use, a treatment should satisfy three criteria: (a) there should be convincing evidence that, compared with no treatment, the treatment is effective in improving health outcomes; (b) compared with no treatment, its beneficial effects on health outcomes should outweigh any harmful effects on health outcomes; (c) compared with the next best alternative treatment, the treatment should represent a good use of resources in the sense that it satisfies principle no. 5.
   ❑ strongly agree ❑ agree ❑ ? ❑ disagree ❑ strongly disagree
   Comment: _____

   _____

10. When making judgments about benefits, harms, and costs, to the greatest extent possible, the judgments should reflect the preferences of the individuals who actually receive the treatments.
    ❑ strongly agree ❑ agree ❑ ? ❑ disagree ❑ strongly disagree
    Comment: _____

    _____

11. When determining whether a treatment satisfies the criteria of principle no. 9, the burden of proof should be on those who want to promote the use of the treatment.
    ❑ strongly agree ❑ agree ❑ ? ❑ disagree ❑ strongly disagree
    Comment: _____

    _____

Review the guidelines for allocation of health care resources that have resulted from this exercise. Would they be helpful to people in your organization in making allocation decisions at various levels, that is from the institutional level to the bedside? If these guidelines fall short of being helpful, what should be done to produce guidelines that are useful?

Do you consider these guidelines to be just? Who would benefit from them? Who would carry the burdens they might impose?

Are these guidelines you would like to see adopted at a national level? What would likely happen if they were widely adopted? Are these the results you would want? Are they fair? What understanding of health care do they seem to promote? Is this acceptable?

Another way to approach the allocation guidelines suggested by Eddy is to take a specific societal or institutional allocation issue and attempt to apply the guidelines (especially #'s 5, 6, 7, and 9), paying particular attention to some of the issues raised in the three paragraphs above.

ENDNOTES

1. Eddy DM. "Three battles to watch in the 1990s." *JAMA.* 1993:270:520-526.

2. Jonsen A. Bentham. "In a box: technology assessment and health care allocation." *Law Med Health Care.* 1986;14:172-174.

3. Eddy DM. "Medicine, money, and mathematics." *Am Coll Surg Bull.* 1992;77:36-49.

4. Eddy DM. "Practice policies: guidelines for methods." *JAMA.* 1990;263:1839-1841.

5. Evidence-Based Medicine Working Group. "Evidence-based medicine: a new approach to teaching the practice of medicine." *JAMA.* 1992;268:2420-2425.

6. Fleming C, Wasson JH, Albertsen PC, Barry MJ, Wennberg JE, for the Prostate Patient Outcomes Research Team. "A decision analysis of alternative treatment strategies for clinically localized prostate cancer." *JAMA.* 1993;269:2650-2568.

7. Eddy DM. "Designing a practice policy: standards, guidelines, and options." *JAMA.* 1990;263:3077, 3081, 3084.

CHAPTER 3

HEALTH REFORM IS DEAD! LONG LIVE HEALTH REFORM!

Uwe E. Reinhardt, Ph.D.

AFTER THE DEMISE OF THE CLINTON HEALTH-REFORM PLAN IN 1994, IT WAS commonly said, "Health reform is dead." That was not an accurate assessment. Health reform is not dead. It is not even half-dead. Rather, half of health reform seems totally dead; the other half is very much alive.

The part that died last year is the decades-old pursuit of the egalitarian dream for American health care, a dream to which politicians of all ideological stripes had hitherto felt compelled to swear allegiance – at least for public consumption. In its place there has come an official embrace of an incomes-based health care system. As trendy newspapers would put it, talk of a one-tiered health system is now "out," and talk of individual managerial and fiscal responsibility for health status and health care (speak: rationing by income class) is "in."

The part of health reform that survived is a veritable revolution in the manner in which health care is produced and sold to American patients. Traditional medical practices, hospitals, pharmacies and other facilities that rendered health care constituted a relatively uncoordinated mosaic of profit centers, whose revenue and income rose when patients were given added services. This system is now being converted into a very tightly coordinated mosaic of cost centers, whose revenue is earned up front in the form of annual capitation payments, and whose income falls when patients are given added services. This revolution is literally standing the traditional economics of health care on its head.

In this essay I shall provide brief commentary on both developments, and offer some speculation on the nature of 21st-century American health care. Because of severe space constraints, the discussion will necessarily be somewhat superficial.[1]

THE NEW SOCIAL CONTRACT IN HEALTH CARE

Whatever one may think of our torturous debate on health reform during the last two years, that debate did settle a decades-old wrestling match over the proper ethical foundation for American health care. For purposes of discussion, one can crystallize this ideological battle by means of a simple, straight-forward question:

To the extent that our health system can make it possible, should the child of a gas-station attendant have the same chance of a healthy life, and the same chance of a cure from a given illness, as does the child of a corporate executive?

If one posed this question to random samples of Canadian or continental-European legislators, the overwhelming majority of them would answer it firmly in the affirmative. (In this respect, the United Kingdom seems the odd one out. It has always been less egalitarian in health care – and in education – than has continental Europe.) These nations' statutes at all levels of government concretely express that view, and their health systems do as well.

If one posed that same question to a random sample of Americans, their answer, for public consumption, probably would be in the affirmative as well. But this nation's laws always have, and probably always will, belie that lofty response. So does the American health system. American legislators, and perhaps the American people as well, simply do not share a common social ethic on the distribution of human services – be it health care or education or justice. If one gave Americans a truth serum and then posed them the question raised above, one would be likely to receive varied responses, rooted in a rather wide ideological spectrum.

At one extreme of that spectrum are the quite sizeable number of Americans who do view health care purely as a social good that is to be shared by all who need it on roughly equal terms, regardless of the individual patient's ability to pay for that care. That view implies the collective financing of health care, strongly guided by the redistributive hand of government. Naturally, this school of thought would answer the question raised above in the affirmative, just as firmly as would continental Europeans and Canadians.

At the other extreme of the spectrum, however, are the apparently quite numerous Americans who view health care as essentially a private consumption good, whose procurement and financing are the individual's responsibility, except perhaps in truly catastrophic cases. Often, but not always, this view is reinforced by the clinical theory that many, if not most, modern diseases are rooted somehow in the individual's own behavior – that illness is not just bad luck beyond the individual's control. This school of thought has been nourished over the years by the writings of libertarian scholars – for example, by the prominent Nobel Laureate economist Milton Friedman, who proposed, in *The Wall Street Journal* of November 19, 1991, that an ideal health insurance policy would be one in which the individual household faces a deductible of $20,000 per year, or 30% of the household's income during the prior two years, which would impose on a family with an annual income of $20,000 per year a deductible of $12,000 per year.

Slightly to the left of the Friedmanesque extreme, but far to the right of the egalitarian school, sits the working majority of the United States Congress (and, possibly, of the American people as well). That majority tends to view health care as similar to other basic commodities, such as food, clothing and shelter. While that ideology does allow that the incidence of some catastrophic illnesses lie totally outside the individual's control, and while it would accord all Americans collectively financed access to at least a basic minimum of critically needed health care in catastrophic cases of illness – regardless of its origin – that school of thought nevertheless countenances a health system that allows the quantity and quality of health care received by individuals to vary systematically by income class, just as the quality of a child's education has traditionally been allowed to vary systematically and quite visibly with the parents' income class (an idea still alien to countries such as Canada or Germany). One may doubt that this school of thought would ever proclaim openly that, to the extent that the health system can make it possible, the child of a corporate executive may legitimately enjoy a better chance of surviving a given illness than the child of a gas-station attendant. Such a proclamation would be political suicide. But, implicitly, the school would countenance precisely that state of affairs.

In the great health-care battle of 1993-94, the "health-care-is-just-like-food" people triumphed over the President and his allies, who had sought with their plan to extract a roughly egalitarian distribution of health care from a market-driven health-care delivery system. It must be said, of course, that in developing their reform plan and in trying to sell it to the Congress and to the American people, the President and his team of advisors made countless tactical (and often tactless) errors that truly astound outsiders who are otherwise well-disposed to the President's social ethic. But surely the President's most serious error was to take the American people at their word when they profess allegiance to an **egalitarian** distribution of health care (or of any other human service, like education or justice). Much of the bureaucratic complexity of the President's plan was driven in large part by his strong emphasis on an egalitarian distribution of health care. It is now clear that Americans will not tolerate either the redistribution of income from the upper to the lower third of the income distribution that would be implied in a more egalitarian health system, nor would they countenance the administrative apparatus necessary to enforce such a redistribution.

Although the "health-care-is-just-like-food" school won its battle squarely, they cannot be said to have won it fairly. Instead of stating their quite legitimate ideology forthrightly, for public scrutiny, they couched it in mellow code words, such as "individual responsibility," "consumer choice," "empowerment," "the freedom to be insured or not," and so on. Anyone able to cut through these code words will quickly realize that they add up to income-based rationing of health care. Practically, all of these code words mean that the preferred American health insurance system is one that empowers well-to-do Americans to allocate their ample budgets between health care and other things as they choose, and that empowers poor Americans to do likewise with their meager income, plus whatever subsidies Congress may or may not bestow on them. It is evident now that these subsidies will range from extremely meager to nothing.

Americans have long looked down on the Canadian and European health systems because, it is said, these nations "ration" health care. There is no doubt that they do, either by the queue or simply by limiting the array of novel technology made available by the health system. Now it is true that, during the past three decades or so, the bulk of well-insured Americans were spared rationing of any sort in health care. For one, the American health system has long been beset by excess capacity all around. In principle, there was no immediate need for rationing access to that abundance. Second, for the well-insured, the financial incentives faced by doctors, hospitals and other providers of health care under the traditional fee-for-service system generously rewarded the unrestrained use of whatever capacity was in place.

For the millions of low-income Americans without health insurance, however, rationing by income and price has always been a fact of life in this country, with well-documented ill consequences for their health.[2] Economists teach their students that the social role of prices is to ration scarce resources among competing wants.[3] On that view, the American health system has rationed health care for at least some Americans all along.

The ideology that triumphed in last year's debate on health care officially sanctions rationing health care by price and income, and it adds another layer to the nation's traditionally two-tiered health system. Henceforth there will be a three-tiered American health system, each with its own rules for rationing health care.

For uninsured Americans who are poor or near-poor – chiefly families of people who work full-time at low wages and salaries – we shall reserve and perhaps expand our current patchwork of public hospitals and clinics. These publicly financed institutions will be sorely underfunded, as they always have been, thus forcing severe limits on their physical capacity. Such limits, in turn, will beget the long queues that have always been the classic instrument of rationing. Lack of funding will also limit the technology available to the physicians working in these public institutions. Honest people will call this budget-driven withholding of technology rationing as well. The uninsured will increasingly be herded into these beleaguered public institutions, because the ever-steeper price discounts extracted from private hospitals by Medicare, Medicaid and private insurers will rob these hospitals of the financial cushion they have hitherto used to finance their charity care.

The employed broad middle class will be enrolled in the newly emerging-health plans, such as health maintenance organizations. These plans will be budgeted prospectively, on a per-capita basis, through competitively bid premiums. To control their outlays, the plans necessarily must limit the patient's choice of doctor and hospital at time of illness. Furthermore, they inevitably will come to withhold some care that patients and their physicians might judge desirable, but that the HMO's management finds too expensive relative to the expected medical benefits. (For example, the cost per "quality-adjusted" life year saved will be judged too high.) Such withholding of care clearly is a form of rationing as well, although one that can be defended, in many instances, on economic grounds.[4]

Finally, for well-to-do Americans there will continue to be the open-ended, free-choice, fee-for-service health system without rationing of any form, even in instances where additional care is of dubious clinical or economic merit. Well-to-do Americans will demand no less, and they will always have it. Furthermore, they will continue to have it on a fully tax-deductible basis, a tax preference to the rich that no economist would ever defend, but that no politician would dare to remove.

America's politically powerful elderly will probably be able to defend their much-cherished, open-ended, free-choice, tax-financed Medicare coverage as well, at least for a while. Alas, theirs is a less certain prospect in the long run. Even before the turn of the century, most of the elderly will probably find themselves enrolled in HMOs as well, at whatever capitation rates the Medicare budget can tolerate under constrained federal spending. In fact, current attempts in the Congress to broach that topic are motivated by the thought that it will be much easier to impose total top-down-budgeting upon capitated premiums than on Medicare's traditional, open-ended, fee-for-service system.

We must leave for study by political scientists whether this politically dominant vision for American health care faithfully reflects the independent preferences of the so-called "grass roots," or whether it merely is being foisted on a bewildered "grass roots" by a small, powerful policy-making elite that knows how to manipulate grass-root "Preferences" through skillfully structured information and outright misinformation. (Some participants in the debate on healthcare reform resorted to the most egregious forms of misinformation on the options before us. In this arena, syndicated columnist George Will's hysterical – and false – assertion that, under the President's plan, Americans who purchase health services deemed unnecessary by government could face a 15-year jail term probably deserves first prize. *Newsweek,* which served as the willing conduit for that misinformation in its issue of February 7, 1994, must share in that dubious prize.) Whatever the case may be, however, we should not delude ourselves any longer that the Congress of the United States will soon contemplate moving us toward the one-tier health system that is still being endorsed officially, by every politician, for public consumption. A case can be made for admitting it openly and for making the quality of the bottom tier the main concern of government health policy, leaving the rest of the system to fend for itself. This will mean strengthening the federal Public Health Service and helping the states in funding their own public health facilities.

THE CONVERSION TO "MANAGED" CARE

In the period from 1960 to 1990, annual health spending in the United States tended to outrun the growth of the non-health component of our Gross National Product (GNP) by about 3 percentage points.[5] On average, if the non-health component of the GNP rose by, say, 7% per year, health spending rose by about 10%. At these trends, health spending would absorb 18% of the GNP by the year 2000, 50% by 2050 and 82% by 2100. Clearly, these trends were not sustainable.

There are basically only two ways to control a nation's spending on health care: 1) regulated fee-for-service compensation, accompanied by indirect controls on the utilization of services and, possibly, by overall budget caps, and 2) capitated managed care, possibly subject to overall budget caps as well.

Under a regulated fee-for-service system, the she individual providers of health care would have faced a predetermined fee schedule – either negotiated or unilaterally set by government. Individual physicians and hospitals would have lost the economic freedom to set their own prices at will, but they generally would have retained the freedom to operate as economically and clinically independent units. Hospitals would have remained free-standing units, and physicians would have remained predominantly self-employed professionals, as they still are in Canada, France and Germany. More importantly, these providers would not have been placed at financial risk for the use of health care by patients. Quite to the contrary, as individual providers they would stand to benefit from added use of health care.

One should have thought that physicians and hospitals would have preferred that approach as the lesser evil of the choice between regulated fee-for-service and capitated managed care. Oddly enough, organized American medicine, for one, had so steadfastly refused even to discuss regulated fee-for-service as an option in the past that inadvertently it surrendered both the economic and the clinical freedom of American physicians straight into the arms of those who write the last check for health care: government, private insurers and the private employers who stand behind those insurers.

These payers will always find a regulated fee-for-advice system cumbersome, mainly because they have so little direct control over the utilization of health care. They are much better off with various forms of top-down budgeting for health care, of which compensation of providers by annual capitation is a prime example. Given the long-standing opposition of physicians and hospitals to regulated fee-for-service – which must have come as a pleasant surprise to these payers – the latter are now in the process of converting the entire health system into what is most aptly described as a form of private-sector "bounty hunting" under which tough, private regulators are enacted with a task that Americans (including physicians and hospital leaders) have been unwilling to entrust to govemment.

In this wild-west scenario of our health sector, doctors, hospitals and the manufacturers of health products have come to play the role of "economic outlaws" whose raids on the treasuries of business and govemment during the 1980s outraged those who pay for health care: government, private employers and patients. Because the sheriff (speak: government) seemed powerless in the face of the raiders – mainly because the sheriff was allowed by the towns-people (speak: payers) to carry only a small caliber gun – the increasingly desperate payers ultimately sought help from a rough bunch of "bounty hunters" the executives of the burgeoning HMO industry. The payers give the "bounty hunters" a flat annual capitation-per-insured-life, along with the license to go after the "economic oudaws" in any way they can, as long as the raids on the payers' treasuries cease and the insured remain satisfied with the health- care received through this process.

The "bounty hunters" carry into this "hunt" a two-barreled shotgun. One barrel consists of the large pools of insured that the "bounty hunters" amass through their marketing blitzes. Merely by threatening to divert parts of these pools from individual doctors, hospitals and health manufacturers, the "bounty hunters" can extract huge price concessions from these frightened providers. That is their bounty. The second barrel consists of the vast computer systems by which the "bounty hunters" monitor and control the doctors and hospitals within their territory, i.e., within their networks. With swift frontier justice, the "bounty hunters" drive from their territory (their list of enrolled providers) any physician, hospital or pharmacist whose statistical practice profile is deemed wanting on clinical or economic grounds.

To be sure, along with the handsome "bounty" earned by the "hunters," their massive advertising campaigns and their micro-management of health care do eat up sizeable chunks of the capitation premiums they collect from business and government – up to 30%. But those chunks are not a new burden on premium payers; they are carved out of the incomes of the providers of health care. The premiums paid by business and government, which rose at double-digit rates in the 1980s, have now been stabilized, and many are even decreasing. From the perspective of patients, taxpayers and private employers, then, competition by means of capitated managed care evidently has been productive, at least so far, and at least insofar as costs are concerned.

That the "hunted" – the doctors, hospitals and other providers of health care – see it differently is not surprising. To them, the emerging market in health care must appear as a veritable siege. While one can have compassion for their current plight, they ought not to be surprised at finding themselves backed into the health-sector's O.K. Corral, so to speak. By steadfastly opposing any other form of cost control for so long they literally invited these private-sector "bounty hunters" onto their turf. Probably their only hope, in the longer run, is to observe the bounty hunters' tactics closely and, eventually, to become bounty hunters themselves – that is, to contract directly with payers, thereby assuming the financial risk for health care of large groups of patients in return for annual capitation payments.

There is, of course, the perennial danger that, after having pocketed their capitation payments up front, the bounty hunters may ride away into the sunset and not deliver to patients all of the care they had promised to deliver in return for their capitation payment. After all, with all revenues received up front, the less the HMOs do for patients in any given year, the more money they get to keep. To preclude that outcome, it will be essential to accompany the conversion to capitated managed care with an external monitoring system capable of providing prospective enrollees with credible information about the experience patients have in competing HMOs. That information must include not only ratings of patients' own satisfaction with their chosen HMO, but also clinical outcomes data that can be understood by, say, experts engaged by employers or governments under whose sponsorship consumers enroll in HMOs. The availability of such credible report cards is crucial to the progress of capitized managed care. It is up to consumers to insist on that information.

CONCLUDING REMARKS

Alas, some innocent bystanders will be hit in the emerging shoot-out at health care's O.K. Corral. The private-sector "bounty hunters" are unlikely to absorb the famous "cost shift" by which charitable doctors and hospitals have hitherto been able to finance catastrophic health insurance for the nation's uninsured simply through higher prices to private payers. But that development may be all for the good. By flushing this chronic social problem into the open, where it can no longer be ignored, the "bounty hunters" may yet force out politicians to confront that problem more forthrightly than they have in the past.

KEY IDEAS IN THIS ARTICLE:

- Health reform is *not* dead. What *is* dead is a key assumption underlying the 1993-94 debate about health care reform: health care is a basic social good that should be available to all on approximately equal terms, despite one's ability to pay.

- A different assumption triumphed in the debate and is shaping current health care reform: health care is one more commodity whose purchase and financing are the individual's responsibility, and whose quantity and quality are very much influenced by income class.

- American legislators, and perhaps the American public as well, do not share a common social ethic on the distribution of human services – be it health care, education, or justice.

- The preferred American health insurance system is one that empowers well-to-do Americans to allocate their ample budgets between health care and other things as they choose, and that empowers poor Americans to do likewise with their meager income, plus whatever subsidies Congress may or may not bestow on them, which are likely to range from extremely meager to nothing.

- A three-tiered system, each with its own implications for rationing health care, will result from this approach. The first tier will consist in the uninsured poor or near-poor, whose care will be rationed through underfunding of public services. The middle class will constitute a second tier, probably enrolled in some form of managed care plan, with its forms of rationing. The third tier will consist in the wealthy, who will continue in a free-choice, fee-for-service arrangement, with essentially no rationing.

- Capitated managed care seems to be successful from the perspective of private employers, insurers, government and even some patients.

- Capitated managed care is not so successful for providers who have lost much economic and clinical freedom.

- One consequence of managed care is the increasing inability of providers to cost-shift in order to provide care for the uninsured.

- The inability to cost-shift may not be entirely bad, for it will finally bring the problem of the un and under-insured into the open, where it can no longer be ignored.

THE ADVANTAGES OF CAPITALISM AND FREE ENTERPRISE

In drawing the distinction between medical care and other commodities on the one hand, and not-for-profit and investor-owned institutions on the other, I am not expressing any general bias against capitalism or the American free enterprise system. We are all beneficiaries of the genius of that system. To paraphrase Pope John Paul II: If by capitalism is meant an economic system which recognizes the fundamental and positive role of business, the market, private property, and the resulting responsibility for the means of production – as well as free human creativity in the economic sector – then its contribution to American society has been most beneficial.

As a key element of the free enterprise system, the American business corporation has proved itself to be an efficient mechanism for encouraging and minimizing commercial risk. It has enabled individuals to engage in commercial activities which none of them could manage alone. In this regard, the purpose of the business corporation is specific: to earn a growing profit and a reasonable rate of return for the individuals who have created it. The essential element here is a *reasonable* rate of return, for without it the commercial corporation cannot exist.

SOCIETY'S NON-ECONOMIC GOODS

That being said, it is important to recognize that not all of society's institutions have as their essential purpose earning a reasonable rate of return on capital. For example, the purpose of the family is to provide a protective and nurturing environment in which to raise children. The purpose of education at all levels is to produce knowledgeable and productive citizens. And the primary purpose of social services is to produce shelter, counseling, food and other programs for people and communities in need. Generally speaking, each of these organizations has as its essential purpose a non-economic goal: the advancement of human dignity.

And this is as it should be. While economics is indeed important, most of us would agree that the value of human life and the quality of the human condition are seriously diminished when reduced to purely economic considerations. Again, to quote Pope John Paul II, the idea that the entirety of social life is to be determined by market exchanges is to run "the risk of an 'idolatry' of the market, an idolatry which ignores the existence of *goods which by their nature are not and cannot be mere commodities*." (Emphasis supplied.)

This understanding is consistent with the American experience. In the belief that the non-economic ends of the family, social services and education are essential to the advancement of human dignity and to the quality of our social and economic life, we have treated them quite differently from most other goods and services. Specifically, we have not made their allocation dependent solely on a person's ability to afford them. For example, we recognize that individual human dignity is enhanced through a good education, and that we all benefit by having an educated society; so we make an elementary and secondary education available to everyone, and heavily subsidize it thereafter. By contrast, we think it quite appropriate that hair spray, compact disks, and automobiles be allocated entirely by their affordability.

HEALTHCARE: NOT SIMPLY A COMMODITY

Now it is my contention that healthcare delivery is one of those "goods which by their nature are not and cannot be mere commodities." I say this because healthcare involves one of the *most* intimate aspects of our lives – our bodies and, in many ways, our minds and spirits as well. The quality of our life, our capacity to participate in social and economic activities, and very often life itself are at stake in each serious encounter with the medical care system. This is why we expect healthcare delivery to be a competent *and* a caring response to the broken human condition – to human vulnerability.

To be sure, we expect our physician to earn a good living and our hospital to be economically viable, but when it comes to *our* case we do not expect them to be motivated mainly by economic self-interest. When it comes to *our* coronary bypass or *our* hip replacement or *our* child's cancer treatment, we expect them to be professional in the original sense of that term – motivated primarily by patient need, not economic self-interest. We have no comparable expectation – nor should we – of General Motors or Wal-Mart. When we are sick, vulnerable and preoccupied with worry, we depend on our physician to be our confidant, our advocate, our guide and agent in an environment that is bewildering for most of us, and where matters of great importance are at stake.

The availability of good healthcare is vital to the character of community life. We would not think well of ourselves if we permitted healthcare institutions to let the uninsured sick and injured go untreated. We endeavor to take care of the poor and the sick as much for our benefit as for theirs. Accordingly, most Americans believe society should provide everyone access to adequate healthcare services just as it ensures everyone an education through grade 12. There is a practical aspect to this aspiration as well, because like education, healthcare entails community-wide needs, which it impacts in various ways: we all benefit from a healthy community, and we all suffer from a lack of health, especially with respect to communicable disease.

Finally, healthcare is particularly subject to what economists call *market failure*. Most healthcare "purchases" are not predictable, nor do medical services come in standardized packages and different grades suitable to comparison shopping and selection – most are specific to individual need. Moreover, it would be wrong to suggest that seriously ill patients defer their healthcare purchases while they shop around for the best price. Nor do we expect people to pay the full cost of catastrophic, financially devastating illnesses. This is why most developed nations spread the risk of these high-cost episodes through public and/or private health insurance. And due to the prevalence of health insurance, or third-party payment, most of us do not pay for our healthcare at the time it is delivered. Thus, we are inclined to demand an infinite amount of the very best care available. In short, healthcare does not lend itself to market discipline in the same way as most other goods and services.

So healthcare – like the family, education, and social services – is *special*. It is fundamentally different from most other goods because it is essential to human dignity and the character of our communities. It is, to repeat, one of those "goods which by their nature are not and cannot be mere commodities." Given this special status, the primary end or essential purpose of medical care delivery should be a cured patient, a comforted patient, and a healthier community, *not* to earn a profit or a return on capital for shareholders. This understanding has long been a central ethical tenet of medicine. The International Code of the World Health Organization, for example, states that doctors must practice their profession "uninfluenced by motives of profit."

THE ADVANTAGES OF NOT-FOR-PROFIT-INSTITUTIONS

This leads me to my second point, that the primary non-economic ends of healthcare delivery are best advanced in a predominantly not-for-profit delivery system.

Before making this argument, however, I need to be very clear about what I am *not* saying. I am *not* saying that not-for-profit healthcare organizations and systems should be shielded from all competition. I believe properly structured competition is good for most not-for-profits. For example, I have long contended that the quality of elementary and secondary education would benefit greatly from the use of vouchers and expanded parental choice in the selection of schools. Similarly, the Catholic Health Association's proposal for healthcare reform envisions organized, economically disciplined healthcare systems competing with one another for enrollees.

Second, I am *not* saying that all not-for-profit hospitals and healthcare systems act appropriately: some do not. But the answer to this problem is greater accountability in their governance and operation, not the extreme measure of abandoning the not-for-profit structure in healthcare.

What I *am* saying is that the not-for-profit structure is the preferred model for delivering healthcare services. This is so because the not-for-profit institution is uniquely designed to provide essential human services. Management expert Peter Drucker reminds us that the distinguishing feature of not-for-profit organizations is not that they are non-profit, but that they do something very different from either business or government. He notes that a business has "discharged its task when the customer buys the product, pays for it, and is satisfied with it," and that government has done so when its "policies are effective." On the other hand, he writes:

> The "non-profit" institution neither supplies goods or services nor controls (through regulation). Its "product" is neither a pair of shoes nor an effective regulation. Its product is a changed human being. The non-profit institutions are human change agents. Their "product" is a cured patient, a child that learns, a young man or woman grown into a self-respecting adult; a changed human life altogether.

In other words, the purpose of not-for-profit organizations is to improve the human condition, that is, to advance important non-economic, non-regulatory functions that cannot be as well served by either the business corporation or government. Business corporations describe success as consistently providing shareholders with a reasonable return on equity. Not-for-profit organizations never properly define their success in terms of profit; those that do have lost their sense of purpose.

This difference between not-for-profits and businesses is most clearly seen in the organizations' different approaches to decision-making. The primary question in an investor-owned organization is: "How do we ensure a reasonable return to our shareholders?" Other questions may be asked about quality and the impact on the community, but always in the context of their effect on profit. A properly focused not-for-profit always begins with a different set of questions:

- What is best for the person who is served?
- What is best for the community?
- How can the organization ensure a prudent use of resources for the whole community, as well as for its intermediate customers?

HEALTHCARE'S ESSENTIAL CHARACTERISTICS

I believe there are four essential characteristics of healthcare delivery that are especially compatible with the not-for-profit structure, but much less likely to occur when healthcare decision-making is driven predominantly by the need to provide a return on equity. These four essential characteristics are:

- access
- medicine's patient-first ethic
- attention to community-wide needs, and
- volunteerism.

Let me discuss each.

First, there is the need for access. Given healthcare's essential relationship to human dignity, society should ensure everyone access to an adequate level of healthcare services. This is why the United States Catholic Conference and I argued strongly last year for universal insurance coverage. This element of healthcare reform remains a moral imperative.

But even if this nation had universal insurance, I would maintain that a strong not-for-profit sector is still critical to access. With primary accountability to shareholders, investor-owned organizations have a powerful incentive to avoid not only the uninsured and underinsured, but also vulnerable and hard-to-serve populations, high-cost populations, undesirable geographic areas, and many low-density rural areas. To be sure, not-for-profits also face pressure to avoid these groups, but *not* with the *added* requirement of generating a return on equity.

Second, not-for-profit healthcare organizations are better suited than their investor-owned counterparts to support the patient-first ethic in medicine. This is all the more important as society moves away from fee-for-service medicine and cost-based reimbursement toward *capitation*. (By "capitation" I mean paying providers in advance a fixed amount per person, regardless of the services required by any specific individual.)

Whatever their economic disadvantages, fee-for-service medicine and cost-based reimbursement shielded the physician and the hospital from the economic consequences of patient treatment decisions and, thereby, provided strong economic support for a patient-first ethic in American medicine. Few insured patients were ever undertreated, though some were inevitably overtreated. Now we face a movement to a fully capitated health-care system which shifts the financial risk in healthcare from the *payers of care* to the *providers*.

This development raises a critically important question: "When the provider is at financial risk for treatment decisions, who is the patient's advocate?" How can we continue to put the patient first in this new arrangement? This challenge will become especially daunting as we move into an intensely price-competitive market, where provider economic survival is on the line everyday. In such an environment, the temptation to undertreat could be significant. Again, not-for-profits will face similar economic pressure, but not with the added requirement of producing a reasonable return on shareholder equity. Part of the answer here, I believe, is to ensure that the nation not convert to a predominantly investor-owned delivery system.

Third, in healthcare there are a host of community-wide needs that are generally unprofitable, and therefore unlikely to be addressed by investor-owned organizations. In some cases, this entails particular services needed by the communty but unlikely to earn a return on investment, such as expensive burn units, neonatal intensive care, or immunization programs for economically deprived populations. Also important are the teaching and research functions needed to renew and advance healthcare.

The community also has a need for continuity and stability of health services. Because the primary purpose of nonprofits is to serve patients and communities, they tend to be deeply rooted in the fabric of the community and are more likely to remain – if they are needed – during periods of economic stagnation and loss. Investor-owned organizations must, on the other hand, either leave the community or change their product line when return-on-equity becomes inadequate.

Fourth, volunteerism and philanthropy are important components of healthcare that thrives best in a not-for-profit setting. As Peter Drucker has noted, volunteerism in not-for-profit organizations is capable of generating a powerful countercurrent to the contemporary dissolution of families and loss of community values. At a time in our history when it is absolutely necessary to strengthen our sense of civic responsibility, volunteerism in healthcare is more important than ever. From the boards of trustees of our premier healthcare organizations to the hands-on delivery of services, volunteers in healthcare can make a difference in peoples' lives and "forge new bonds to community, a new commitment to achieve citizenship, to social responsibility, to values."

ROLE OF MEDIATING INSTITUTIONS

In addition to my belief that the not-for-profit structure is especially well-aligned with the central purpose of healthcare, let me suggest one more reason why each of us should be concerned that not-for-profits remain a vibrant part of the nation's healthcare delivery system: They are important *mediating institutions*.

The notion of mediating structures is deeply rooted in the American experience. On the one hand, these institutions stand between the individual and the state; on the other, they mediate against the rougher edges of capitalism's inclination toward excessive individualism. Mediating structures, such as family, church, education and healthcare, are the institutions closest to the control and aspirations of most Americans.

The need for mediating institutions in healthcare is great. Private sector failure to provide adequately for essential human services, such as healthcare, invites government intervention. While government has an obligation to ensure the availability of and access to essential services, it generally does a poor job of delivering them. Wherever possible, we prefer that government work through and with institutions that are closer and more responsive to the people and communities being served. This role is best played by not-for-profit hospitals. Neither public nor private, they are the heart of the voluntary sector in healthcare.

Earlier, I identified several reasons why I believe investor-owned organizations are not well-suited to meeting all of society's needs and expectations regarding healthcare. Should the investor-owned entity ever become the predominant form of healthcare delivery, I believe that our country will inevitably experience a sizeable and substantial growth in government intervention and control.

Until now, I have made two arguments: first, that healthcare is more than a commodity – it is a service essential to human dignity and to the quality of community life; and second, that the not-for-profit structure is best aligned with this understanding of healthcare's primary mission. My concluding argument is that private and public sector leaders have an urgent civic responsibility to preserve and strengthen our nation's predominantly not-for-profit healthcare delivery system.

This is a pressing obligation because the not-for-profit sector in healthcare may already be eroding as a result of today's extremely turbulent competitive environment in healthcare. The problem, let me be clear, is *not* competition per se, but the kind of competition that undermines healthcare's essential mission and violates the very character of the not-for-profit organization by encouraging it – even requiring it – to behave like a commercial enterprise.

Contemporary healthcare markets are characterized by hospital overcapacity and competition for scarce primary care physicians, but also and more ominously by shrinking health insurance coverage, and growing risk selection in private health insurance markets. These latter two features encourage health-care providers to compete by becoming very efficient at avoiding the uninsured and high-risk populations, and by reducing necessary but unprofitable community services – behavior that strikes at the heart of the not-for-profit mission in healthcare. Moreover, the environment leads some healthcare leaders to conclude that the best way to survive is to become for-profit or to create for-profit subsidiaries. The existence of not-for-profits is further threatened by the aggressive efforts of some investor-owned chains to expand their market share by purchasing not-for-profit hospitals and by publicly challenging the continuing need for not-for-profit organizations in healthcare.

ADVANCING THE NOT-FOR-PROFIT HEALTHCARE MISSION

Each of us and our communities have much to lose if we allow unstructured market forces to continue to erode the necessary and valuable presence of not-for-profit healthcare organizations. It is imperative, therefore, that we immediately begin to find ways to protect and strengthen them.

How can we do this? Without going into specifics, I believe it will require a combination of private sector and governmental initiatives. Voluntary hospital board members and executives must renew their institutions' commitment to the essential mission of not-for-profit healthcare. Simultaneously, government must reform health insurance markets to prevent "redlining" and assure everyone reasonable access to adequate healthcare services. Finally, government should review its tax policies to ensure that existing laws and regulations are not putting not-for-profits at an inappropriate competitive disadvantage, but are holding them strictly accountable for their tax exempt status.

Let me conclude by simply reiterating the thesis I made at the beginning of this talk. Healthcare is fundamentally different from most other goods and services. It is about the most human and intimate needs of people, their families, and communities. It is because of this critical difference that each of us should work to preserve the predominantly not-for-profit character of our healthcare delivery in Chicago and throughout the country.

BIBLIOGRAPHY

Bernardin, Joseph L. "The Consistent Ethic of Life and Health Care Reform," *Origins*: vol. 24, June 9, 1994, pp. 60-64.

Dougherty, Charles J. "The Costs of Commercial Medicine," *Theoretical Medicine*: vol. 11, 1990, pp. 275-286.

John Paul II "Centesimus Annus," *Origins*: vol. 21, May 16, 1991, pp. 1-24.

Relman, Arnold S. "What Market Values Are Doing to Medicine," *The Atlantic Monthly*: March 1992, pp. 99-106.

KEY IDEAS IN THIS ARTICLE:

- A good society needs both economic goods (cars, toasters, computers, etc.) and non-economic goods (families, education, healthcare, etc.). It should treat these different goods in essentially different ways.

- There are two different kinds of social institutions: 1) those whose primary purpose is to earn a profit and reasonable rate of return on investment; 2) those whose primary purpose is to advance human dignity (family, schools, courts, cities, etc.).

- "The idea that the entirety of social life is to be determined by market exchanges is to run 'the risk of an idolatry of the market, an idolatry which ignores the existence of goods which, by their nature, are not and cannot be mere commodities.' "

- "The purpose of a not-for-profit organization is to improve the human condition, that is to advance important non-economic, non-regulatory functions that cannot be as well-served by either business corporations or government."

- "The primary question in an investor-owned organization is: how do we ensure a reasonable return to our shareholders? Other questions may be asked . . . but always in the context of their effect on profit."

- Four essential characteristics of healthcare delivery are especially compatible with not-for-profit structure:

  a) Access: "With primary accountability to shareholders, investor-owned organizations have a powerful incentive to avoid uninsured . . . hard-to-serve, high-cost populations . . . undesirable geographic . . . low-density rural areas."

  b) Patient-first ethic: "Not-for-profit healthcare organizations are better-suited than their investor-owned counterparts to support the patient-first ethic in medicine."

  c) Community-wide needs: "In healthcare, there are a host of community-wide needs that are generally unprofitable, and therefore unlikely to be addressed by investor-owned organizations."

  d) Volunteerism: "Volunteerism and philanthropy are important components of healthcare that thrive best in a not-for-profit setting."

- Besides business and government, we need mediating institutions (e.g., family, church, schools, healthcare facilities). Such institutions stand between large, bureaucratic government and the individual; they also mediate against the rougher edges of capitalism's inclination toward excessive individualism. The character of not-for-profit healthcare is more compatible with effective mediating institutions.

- "Private and public sector leaders have an urgent civic responsibility to preserve and strengthen our nation's predominantly not-for-profit healthcare delivery system."

A SUGGESTED PROCESS FOR REFLECTING ON THIS ARTICLE:

(See pages 234-254 for other processes that might better fit your specific goals and objectives.)

A few key ideas could be selected to provide a sharper focus and more in-depth discussion of the issues. For example, ideas 1-5 might be selected. The focus could be in the area of intellectual understanding and agreement.

1. A good society needs both economic goods (cars, toasters, computers, etc.) and non-economic goods (families, education, healthcare, etc.). It should treat these different goods in essentially different ways.

   What makes sense to me about this is:

   What does not make sense to me about this is:

2. There are two different kinds of social institutions: 1) those whose primary purpose is to earn a profit and reasonable rate of return on investment; 2) those whose primary purpose is to advance human dignity (family, schools, courts, cities, etc.).

   What makes sense to me about this is:

   What does not make sense to me about this is:

3. "The idea that the entirety of social life is to be determined by market exchanges is to run 'the risk of an idolatry of the market, an idolatry which ignores the existence of goods which by their nature are not and cannot be mere commodities.' "

   What makes sense to me about this is:

   What does not make sense to me about this is:

4. "The purpose of a not-for-profit organization is to improve the human condition, that is to advance important non-economic, non-regulatory functions that cannot be as well-served by either business corporations or government."

   What makes sense to me about this is:

   What does not make sense to me about this is:

5. "The primary question in an investor-owned organization is: how do we ensure a reasonable return to our shareholders? Other questions may be asked . . . but always in the context of their effect on profit."

   What makes sense to me about this is:

   What does not make sense to me about this is:

IN LIGHT OF OUR DISCUSSION:

- as (executive committee, ethics committee, etc.), what are some next steps that we should take?

- as (hospital, home health agency, etc.), what are some next steps that we should take?

- what systems and structures call for special attention in order to improve the situation?

CHAPTER 5

THE ETHICS OF EXCESS

Richard D. Lamm, LLB CPA

MY WIFE HAD BREAST CANCER IN 1981, WHICH WAS DISCOVERED BY A mammogram. After her (successful) mastectomy, we made a practice of helping dedicate any mammography machine anywhere in Colorado. We were grateful and wanted to help expand this important service and, of course, every hospital loved to have either the Governor or the First Lady at their dedication.

In 1991, however, a study in the *Annals of Internal Medicine*[1] showed that although America had 10,000 mammography machines, we essentially utilized 2600 of them. The study posited out that if every woman had a mammogram every time the American Cancer Association suggested it was appropriate, we would utilize approximately 5000 – still half as many as were then in existence. The study further showed that because the underutilized machines had to be amortized, American women had to pay more than twice what the real cost was, and this was having the effect of driving American women away from mammograms. It also found sites that did not do a sufficient number of mammograms had more flawed readings of the results. Welcome to the new world of excess preventing access and quality. (There are now 16,000 mammography machines in the United States, six times as many as are fully utilized.)

Recognizing that you can never have perfect utilization, and such formulas are thus not perfect, the fact remains – in the case of mammography machines, as elsewhere in the health care system – that excess is interfering with access.

I am increasingly disturbed by the number of well-intentioned people making what they think are health-producing decisions who are, in fact, adding duplicative, superfluous health care facilities to the system. The net effect of these actions has been to build a great redundancy into our health care system, at the same time great need exists in other parts of the system. Half-empty hospitals exist blocks from where children lack access to vaccinations. We have trained far too many medical specialists. Yet, a few streets away from every medical center, women go without prenatal care. Excess sits cheek-to-jowl with inadequacy.

I suggest the sheer magnitude of this problem has become an ethical one. We are all trustees of the U.S. health care system – whatever our roles.

We must eventually take responsibility for the indirect as well as the direct consequences of our actions. A hospital administrator in Colorado, which has a statewide hospital occupancy of less than 50%,[2] cannot say that the 500,000 uninsured Coloradans have nothing to do with his/her facility. That facility is consuming significant resources which are desperately needed elsewhere in the system.

Once a community, state, or nation builds up a medical infrastructure, it must pay for that infrastructure. If it is too large, the citizens pay too much. The Government Accounting Office (GAO) has found:

> Health spending per capita increases with the size of a state's health infrastructure, with hospital and physicians' services accounting for approximately two-thirds of the total personal health spending. States with greater health resources, including physicians as well as hospital and nursing home beds, have higher health care spending on the average.[3]

Supply seems to drive demand and create its own demand. Boston has twice as many hospitals per capita as New Haven, and it has twice as many hospital admissions with *no* difference in outcome.

> A 50% increase in the capacity of the acute hospital sector decreases the threshold for admitting patients in a way that results in a 50% increase in hospital use.[4a]

The number of specialists often determines how many and what types of procedures are performed in the community. The biggest correlation to the number of tonsillectomies, prostatectomies, hysterectomies, and hernia repairs is not the underlying health of the population, but the number of specialists in the area. Rates for appendectomies, which is not an elective procedure, are nearly geographically uniform, while elective procedures, where doctors have discretion, vary by disturbing amounts. The major determinant of how many procedures are done in a given area is the number of specialists in the area who can perform them.[1,5,6] One expert captured the dynamics perfectly:

> . . . in order to gain competitive advantage, there are strong economic incentives for providers to develop new, state-of-the-art facilities and services. This kind of development, in turn, encourages unnecessary or inappropriate utilization in order to generate sufficient revenue to cover the operating and capital costs of the new capacity.[7]

Much of what we do in health care serves the interests of the physician or a particular institution rather than the interests of the public. Well-meaning people continually turn away from facing the ethical implications of this dynamic.

EXCESS PHYSICIANS

There have been a number of studies[8] that have found that America is training too many physicians. These studies generally point out that training too many physicians can be as big a mistake as training too few. The medical profession has ignored report after report showing that it was training too many physicians. And it is clearly expensive. Ginzberg speculates:

> If we would have increased physicians from 140 per 100,000 (1962) to 190 per 100,000 (1990) instead of the 250 per 100,000 which actually occurred, potential savings would amount to $173 billion out of the health spending of $660 billion.[9]

The Bureau of Health Professions estimates that the United States currently has 15,000 surplus physicians; and by the year 2000, they will have 50,000 surplus physicians There are other estimates which put this number considerably higher. Currently, we do know that America has 240 physicians per 100,000 people; and by the year 2000, our 126 medical schools will raise that number to 260 per 100,000 people.[11,12]

On the other hand, Health Maintenance Organizations (HMOs) – one of the main models for managed competition – operate at 120 doctors per 100,000 subscribers.[13] Fee-for-service medicine commonly uses 450 to 500 doctors per 100,000 people,[14] but society is demanding more efficiency and is experimenting with 17 varieties of restructured delivery systems that will dramatically multiply the effectiveness of each physician.

Kissick at the University of Pennsylvania estimates that if we could serve all of America with the same efficiency that Kaiser Permanente serves its system, we would need less than half the number of existing physicians.[15] In the face of clear evidence, U.S. medical schools should dramatically reduce the number of physicians they train, while in fact they actually increased the number. "Cost containment may ultimately require constraints on the number of physicians allowed to enter the system," says John Hughes of Yale University School of Medicine.[12] Recognizing that one cannot serve rural America with the same efficiency as Kaiser serves its subscribers (Kaiser's demography is somewhat different also), Kissick suggests this comparison clearly shows that America will experience tremendous dislocation among physicians, as Adam Smith restructures the marketplace and more and more physicians go to work in groups or for salaries in large systems.[16] Those physicians unwilling or unable to make an arrangement with a health care system will be forced to go to a rural or inner city area, retire, or leave the practice of medicine. Many specialists will seek retraining in the growth sector of primary care.

There is other evidence of this surplus. The Medical Economics Continuing Survey finds that 45% of doctors reported they were not practicing at their full capacity.[16] All the empirical evidence we have confirms that America has too many physicians and that this problem will grow worse before it gets better.

Specialists

We have not only trained too many doctors, we have trained the wrong types.[18-20] Simply stated, other developed industrial countries for many years have practiced medicine with roughly 50% of physicians in primary care and 50% in specialties and subspecialties.[18-20] In the United States, however, we train and employ about 32% primary care physicians (such as general practitioners, family physicians, general internists, general pediatricians, and some obstetrician/gynecologists and emergency medicine physicians), and about 68% specialists and subspecialists.[18-20] Other developed countries, however, do as well or better than the United States at providing care at much lower cost (whether cost is measured as the amount per capita per year, or as a percentage of the GNP). Yet, the situation in the United States is rapidly getting worse. The percentage of physicians graduating from U.S. medical schools who are declaring generalist fields has drastically declined during the last decade, from 36% of the graduating class of 1982 to only 14% in 1992.[18-20]

Comparing the 50:50 specialist-to-generalist ratio desired and the existing 68:32 ratio, one finds a shortfall of approximately 100,000 generalist physicians and an oversupply of 100,000 specialists and subspecialist physicians.[21-23] Compounding this excess, existing models of managed care show that if the federal government, individual states, or the private marketplace create health alliances or accountable health partnerships for everyone, we will need a work force that more closely approximates a 35% specialist and 65% generalist physician distribution, according to Sokolov. Using such models and some basic arithmetic, one can demonstrate a shortfall of 200,000 generalist physicians between current physician supply and what may be needed in the near future. The Pew Health Professions Commission did not accept the number, but it did the trend. Few people argue that we do not have too many specialists.

Wennberg has made a similar analysis:

> If the hiring practices of prepaid group practice HMOs had been in force throughout the United States in 1988, more than half of all specialists would now be unemployed.[4b]

He further adds:

> . . . if radiology residency programs were completely eliminated, it would still take about twenty years before the numbers per capita in the national economy approached the numbers now hired by prepaid group practice HMOs. Under the same policy, it would take more than twenty-five years for the supply of neurosurgeons and about seventeen years for the supply of urologists to approximate the numbers employed by these HMOs.[4c]

An example of the excess in specialties is found in a recent study by Leape, where he looked at the number of surgeons in the United States has compared to what is likely to be needed under the new health care delivery systems. He pointed out that the AMA projected the total supply of surgeons will increase 14% between 1986 and 2010, with most of the growth occurring in surgical specialties. Using productivity standards that are widely agreed upon, he finds that half of the surgeons in the United States are presently significantly underutilized. He points out that staff model HMOs use surgeons two or even three times more efficiently than fee-for-service medicine.[24] At the same time, they perform significantly fewer operations. Fewer surgeons will, in the future, perform fewer operations and yet produce more health.

Medical Schools

In the face of clear evidence, U.S. medical schools should dramatically reduce the number of physicians they train. If America comes anywhere near achieving the efficiency of an HMO in its entire health care system, there will be no need for medical schools to turn out approximately 16,000 physicians a year. An unneeded medical school is an expensive luxury, which cannot be tolerated in an efficient system.

The remaining medical schools should recognize that they have an ethical obligation to dramatically increase the number of primary care physicians they graduate, and to reduce the number of specialists. Supply and demand have never heretofore been a concern to medical schools. As a tragic result, a generation of young professionals are being prepared, at great public and personal expense, for careers where employment will be limited and perhaps not even available. Left unchanged, in fact, the 25 billion public dollars we devote to training health professionals will give our society professionals we simply do not need.

The future system will require medical schools to take much more into consideration the community needs for health manpower, and require them to match their output to what the market needs.

Recognizing that there are many rural and inner-city areas which are not adequately served by doctors, one nevertheless has to predict that there will be a considerable surplus of doctors after health care reform takes effect. This conclusion is reached after looking at a number of comparisons with other health care organizational models.

EXCESS INSTITUTIONAL CAPACITY

It is axiomatic that a nation must pay for its medical infrastructure. Once a hospital is built, or a doctor trained, or a piece of medical technology put in place, it almost inevitably has to be funded. America has too much health care infrastructure that is draining too many dollars from other important needs. This costs America dearly.

Hospital Beds

Most industrialized nations put strict limits on hospitals, hospital beds, and medical technology. European countries seem to recognize that once hospital beds are in place and once doctors and specialists have graduated, they will be used. There is a Parkinson's Law to hospital beds and medical technology: *The work expands to fill facilities available.* Even though the United States actually has a smaller number of hospital beds per capita than most nations, we deliver by far the most intensive treatment while in that bed. We may have fewer beds per capita than other countries, but our beds are often dramatically underoccupied, and a large number of patients in a hospital do not really need to be there. The United States averages 3.8 hospital beds per 1,000 people.[2a] Yet, some experts estimate that because of outpatient surgery, drug therapy, and other medical advances, we only need 1.8 beds per 1,000 people.[13] We have massive underutilized capacity in most metropolitan areas. The United States seems to have a "7-11" theory of hospitals, where we want a hospital on every corner filled with every marvelous machine and open 24 hours a day. This is a terribly expensive luxury – one we can no longer afford.

Excess capacity creates its own demand. Health economists have an axiom, called Roemer's Law, which states: "A built bed is a filled bed." Not totally true, of course, but a built bed is a magnet that does create demand. As Evans has noted:

> . . . overall bed capacity emerges from study after study as the single most important factor influencing hospital inpatient utilization, and the level of bed capacity at which use would appear to stop responding to increases is double or triple current capacity or need estimates.[26]

At any given time, approximately one-third of America's 924,040 staffed hospital beds are empty.[27] This is staffed beds – licensed beds are actually a much higher figure. Large HMOs in the United States operate with only 1.5 beds per 1,000 members.[13] Put another way, HMOs operate with less than half the hospital beds per capita as now exist, and yet keep their subscribers every bit as healthy as fee-for-service medicine.

America may have over 1000 unnecessary surplus hospitals, which think they are contributing to the nation's health, but actually consume resources desperately needed elsewhere in the system.

> "There is clearly excess capacity in the system," says Richard Wade, spokesman for the American Hospital Association. He predicts 20% to 25% hospital capacity will be cut, along with many of the 3.5 million people employed in hospitals. In 1992, 39 of the country's 5,000 hospitals closed with many more shrinking their staff.[28]

Of course, many uninsured will be brought into the US. health care system; but since many of them are already inefficiently served in emergency rooms, this is unlikely to save the large scale closure of hospitals.

Centers of Excellence

America has 850 hospitals doing open heart surgery;[29] less than half do the minimum number (250) to meet federal standards. A hundred of these hospitals do less than one heart surgery a week. Under an efficient health care system, many of these institutions will close. There is no way, for instance, that the Denver metropolitan area needs 14 open heart surgeries,[30] or that Colorado needs four hospitals doing heart transplants. HMOs either own their hospitals or contract with one highly efficient hospital. If America follows the experience of European countries, it will close some of its redundant hospitals, and create centers of excellence which consolidate specific operations in specialized centers.

Intensive Care Beds

It is estimated that $62 billion of the $809 billion of health care in 1992 was for the expense of intensive care units.[31,32] The United States has approximately three times more intensive care beds as do other developed countries. For instance, our intensive care unit (ICU) utilization is 2.5 times that of Canada.[31,33] Whereas 8% of the total Canadian inpatient costs were allocated to ICU units, the United States had 20% of its inpatient care costs allocated to ICU units. Intensive care units employ about 19% of the nurses who worked in general specialty bed units.[31]

The reason that the United States has so many more intensive care beds is that we have different standards about who we put in an intensive care bed. By the standards of other nations, we put many people into an intensive care bed for whom there is no happy outcome. And, conversely, we often put people in an intensive care bed who are not sick enough to really need such a level of care. Eight percent of patients in intensive care units consume 92% of the inpatient hospital resources; and of those 8% high-cost patients, 70% died in the hospital.[31-33] It would seem clear from the statistics that other developed countries with very similar standards and culture with regard to death and dying are much more thoughtful about the categories of people who have access to an intensive care bed.[30-33] In America, we expend massive resources often only to give someone an expensive death.

THE MYTH OF MEDICAL TECHNOLOGY

Americans love technology of any type. Much of this is justified and has led to our being a world leader in the manufacture and use of technology. It is deeply ingrained into our culture. But there is a widespread belief that *medical* technology saves money. Alas, it does not. Here's what one study found on medical technology:

> . . . most technological innovations in the health service industry have added to, rather than reduced costs. This *added* cost reflects a qualitative difference in what the client receives. For example, today's treatment for a particular ailment will almost certainly include a set of therapeutic procedures that is markedly different from what would have been received 25 years ago. . . . In short, the question is not whether recent technological developments have added to health costs. They have. The real question is whether the benefits exceed the costs, and in at least some instances, they may not.[31-33]

Some critics question whether hospitals actually add technology to save health care costs. Evans observes:

> Technological innovations that really reduce costs, simultaneously and by definition, reduce sales and income as well. That is not the end most health providers seek when adding a new technology.[34]

Newhouse, an economist at Harvard, estimates that half of the increase in the national bill for medical care now goes to pay for new technology.[35] Whatever the motivation, medical technology does not come cheap and seldom saves money. Our miracles are often very expensive.

The United States has far more medical technology than it can effectively utilize. With 4.7% of the world's population, we have one-half of the world's CT scanners, and about two-thirds of the world's magnetic resonance imagers (MRIs). In 1987, the United States had 7.4 times as many radiation therapy units and 8 times as many MRIs per million people as did Canada, and had 4.4 times as many open heart surgery units and 2.8 times as many lithotripter units as did Germany.[36]

The state of Colorado has 22 stationary MRIs in hospitals – three on the same block in Denver.[37] Although Canada has the same number of MRIs as Colorado, Canada has nine times our population. Colorado has a myriad of un-met social needs. Yet, it is wasting resources on duplicative, redundant medical technology that often exists in a hospital which is itself not needed for the health of the state.

CONCLUSION

I would suggest that the sheer size of the health care system has become an ethical issue. It is filled with highly trained (and highly paid) people who believe they are adding to the nation's health. Often they are not. They are utilizing resources desperately needed elsewhere in the system. The opportunity costs of those resources could go a long way toward correcting the inadequacies in the system. Excess is interfering with access, and ethical people should work to correct both.

Mr. Lamm was Governor of Colorado from 1975 to 1987. He is currently Director of the Center for Public Policy & Contemporary Issues, University of Denver and Chairman for the Pew Health Professions Commission.

KEY IDEAS IN THIS ARTICLE:

- The American health care system is characterized by excess: there are too many hospitals with too many beds; too many physicians currently and too many being trained; an excess of specialists and sub-specialists with not enough primary care physicians; more medical schools than are needed; too much duplication of services within the same area (e.g., cardiac surgery); too many ICU beds that are too often used for patients who are not sick enough or too sick to benefit; too much medical technology, which all too often is redundant in a given area.

- This excess prevents access and quality. The more there is, the greater the cost to maintain it and the greater the incentive to use it. Both in turn lead to higher costs. These costs are born by taxpayers and patients, and the high costs of health care (higher than they need to be because of the excess) deter many individuals from pursuing needed services. Furthermore, the excess stands in stark contrast to appalling paucity, e.g., women without prenatal care, children without vaccinations.

- The size of American health care is itself an ethical issue.

- Highly trained and highly paid individuals within the health care system are utilizing resources desperately needed elsewhere in the system.

- Opportunity costs of those resources could go a long way toward correcting the inadequacies of the system.

- Ethical people should work to correct both excess and access.

A SUGGESTED PROCESS FOR REFLECTING ON THIS ARTICLE:

(See pages 234-254 for other processes that might better fit your specific goals and objectives.)

	What Makes Sense	What Doesn't Make Sense	Issues/ Implications for Public Policy	Issues/ Implications for Our Locality
The infrastructure of the American health care system is characterized by excess.				
This excess prevents access and quality.				
Costs of infrastructure resources could go a long way to correct the inadequacies of the system.				

ENDNOTES

1. Is the supply of mammography machines outstripping need and demand? Ann Intern Med 1990;113:547

2. Facts about Colorado hospitals. Denver. Colorado Hospital Assn 1991:1-2.

3. State health care spending factors. Publication No. B-2446979. Washington DC: Government Accounting Office, 1992; Feb. 13.

4. Wennberg et al. *Health Affairs* 1993 12(2):(a) 94; (b) 95; (c) 97.

5. Schroeder SA. Health care reform: a special report. *Med Econ.* New York. 1993, p. 32.

6. Phelps C, Health economics. New York. Harper-Collins, 1993.

7. Coddington D et al. The crisis in health care. Jossey-Bass 1990:6.

8. Pew Health Professions Commission staff report. 1993.

9. Ginzberg E. *JAMA* 1992 Feb. 2.

10. Improving access to health care through physician workforce reforms: dimensions for the 21st century. New York. Council on Graduate Medical Education, October 1992.

11. Rising health care costs: causes, implications, and strategies. Congressional Budget Office Washington, DC: April 1991, p. xii.

12. Hughes JS. *Wall Street J,* 1991 May 8, Sect B:I.

13. World development report. The World Bank 1993, chap. 6, p. 6.

14. Reinhardt UE. Health manpower forecasting: the case of physician supply. In E Ginzberg, editor. Health services research: key to health policy. Cambridge: Harvard University Press, 1991.

15. Schroeder SA. Physician supply in the U.S. medical market place. *Health Affairs*, spring 1992, p. 235.

16. Kissick WL. Medicine's dilemmas. New Haven: Yale University Press 1994.

17. Owens A. How low can productivity go? *Med Econ* 1987:64 (25) 172-203.

18. Petersdorf RD. The doctor is in. Washington, DC: Association of American Medical Colleges, 1993.

19. Levinsky NG. Recruiting for primary care. *N Engl J Med* 1993:328:656-60.

20. Politzer R, Harris DL, Gaston MH, and Mullan F. Primary care physician supply and the underserved. *JAMA* 1991: 266: 104-109.

21. Council on Graduate Medical Education. Improving access to health care through physician workforce reform: directions for the 21st century. Rockville (MD): Health Resources and Services Administration, Public Health Service October 1992.

22. Lundberg GD and Lamm RD. Solving our primary care crisis by retraining specialists to gain specific primary care competencies. *JAMA* 1993:270(3):380-381.

23. Lundberg GD. Caring for the uninsured and underinsured. *JAMA* 1991:266:2079-2080.

24. Leape LL. The future of surgery. In RJ Blendon and TS, Hyams eds. Reforming the system: containing health care costs in an era of universal coverage. 1992: p. 213.

25. Roemer M. Bed supply and hospital utilization: a natural experiment. *J Am Hosp Assn* 1961:35:36-42.

26. Evans RG. Strained mercy. Butterworthy 1984.

27. Inglehart J. The American health care system. *N Engl J Med* 1993: July 29, 372.

28. Wade R. *Wall Street J* 1993: July 13, Sect A:2.

29. Medicare tries to save with one fee billing. *Wall Street J* 1992: Sect. A-1.

30. Excess capacity. Report. Rocky Mountain Health Institute 1991: Dec. 7.

31. Schapera DV, et 21 Intensive care: survival and expense of treating critically ill cancer patients. *JAMA* 1993:269:783-786.

32. Jacobs, Roseworthy. *Crit Care Med* 1990: November vol. 13:11.

33. Siro CA et al. An initial comparison of intensive care in Japan and the U.S. *Crit Care Med* 1992:20:1207.

34. Evans RF,. Illusions of necessity: evading responsibility for choices in health care. *J Health Polit Policy Law* fall 1985:10:453.

35. Newhouse, J. New York Times 1993: March 21, Sect F:5.

36. Cordes S. The economics of health service. Cooperative Extension Service, Pennsylvania State University.

37. Aaron HJ. Serious and unstable condition: financing America's health care. Brookings Institute 1991: p. 86.

38. Division of Shortage Designation. Rockville, MD: Bureau of Health Care Delivery and Assistance, Public Health Service, 1992.

CHAPTER 6

REFRAMING THE DEBATE ON HEALTH CARE REFORM BY REPLACING OUR METAPHORS

George J. Annas, J.D., M.P.H.

METAPHORS MATTER, AS OUR STERILE DEBATE ON THE FINANCING OF health insurance demonstrates so well. In that debate the traditional metaphor of American medicine, the military metaphor, was displaced by the market metaphor in public discourse. Metaphors, which entice us to understand and experience "one kind of thing in terms of another . . . play a central role in the construction of social and political reality."[1] The market metaphor proved virtually irresistible in the public arena and led Congress to defer to market forces to "reform" the financing of health insurance in the United States.

We live in a country founded on the proposition that we are all endowed by our creator with certain inalienable rights, especially the rights to life, liberty and the pursuit of happiness. Any government-sponsored health care plan must take into account the assumption by Americans that these rights support entitlement to whatever makes them happy. Perhaps equally important, we live in a wasteful, technologically driven, individualistic and death-denying culture. Every health care plan, government-sponsored or not, must also take these postmodern American characteristics into account. How is it even possible to think seriously about reforming a health care system that reflects these primal and pervasive American values and characteristics? I believe the first necessary step – which will require us to look deeper than money and means, to goals and ends – is to devise a new metaphor to frame our discussion of public policy and to help us develop a new conception of health care. We have tried the military metaphor and the market metaphor; both narrow our field of vision, and neither can take us where we need to go.

THE MILITARY METAPHOR

The military metaphor has had a pervasive influence on both the practice and the financing of medicine in the United States, perhaps because until recently, most U.S. physicians had served in the military. Examples are legion.[2,3] Medicine is a battle against death. Diseases attack the body, and physicians intervene. We are almost constantly engaged in wars on various diseases, such as cancer and AIDS. Physicians, who are mostly specialists backed by allied health professionals and trained to be aggressive, fight these invading diseases with weapons designed to knock them out. Physicians give orders in the trenches and on the front lines, using their armamentaria in search of breakthroughs. Treatments are conventional or heroic, and the brave patients soldier on. We engage in triage in the emergency department, invasive procedures in the operating theater, and even defensive medicine when a legal enemy is suspected.

The military metaphor leads us to overmobilize and to think of medicine in terms that have become dysfunctional. For example, this perspective encourages us to ignore costs, and prompts hospitals and physicians to engage in medical arms races in the belief that all problems can be solved with more sophisticated technology. The military metaphor also leads us to accept as inevitable organizations that are hierarchical and dominated by men. It suggests that viewing the patient's body as a battlefield is appropriate, as are short-term, single-minded tactical goals. Military thinking concentrates on the physical, sees control as central, and encourages the expenditure of massive resources to achieve dominance.

As pervasive as the military metaphor is in medicine, the metaphor itself has been so sanitized that it is virtually unrelated to the reality of war. We have not, for example, used the metaphor to assert that medicine, like war, should be financed and controlled only by the government. The metaphor has also become mythic.[4] As a historian of war, John Keegan, correctly argues, modern warfare has become so horrible that "it is scarcely possible anywhere in the world today to raise a body of reasoned support for the opinion that war is a justifiable activity."[5]

THE MARKET METAPHOR

The market metaphor has already transformed the way we think about fundamental relations in medical care, but is just as dysfunctional as the military metaphor. In the language of the market, for example, health plans and hospitals market products to consumers, who purchase them on the basis of price. Medical care is a business that necessarily involves marketing through advertising and competition among suppliers, who are primarily motivated by profit. Health care becomes managed care. Mergers and acquisitions become core activities. Chains are developed, vertical integration is pursued, and antitrust worries proliferate. Consumer choice becomes the central theme of the market metaphor.[6] In the language of insurance, consumers become "covered lives" (or even "money-generating biological structures"[7]). Economists become health-financing gurus. The role of physicians is radically altered as they are instructed by managers that they can no longer be patient advocates (but instead must advocate for the entire group of covered lives in the health plan). The goal of medicine becomes a healthy bottom line instead of a healthy population.

The market metaphor leads us to think about medicine in already familiar ways: emphasis is placed on efficiency, profit maximization, customer satisfaction, the ability to pay, planning, entrepreneurship, and competitive models.

The ideology of medicine is displaced by the ideology of the marketplace.[8,9] Trust is replaced by *caveat emptor*. There is no place for the poor and uninsured in the metaphor of the market. Business ethics supplant medical ethics as the practice of medicine becomes corporate. Nonprofit medical organizations tend to be corrupted by adopting the values of their for-profit competitors. A management degree becomes at least as important as a medical degree. Public institutions, which by definition cannot compete in the for-profit arena, risk demise, second-class status, or simply privatization.

Like the military metaphor, the market metaphor is also a myth. Patients, as consumers, are to make decisions, but these decisions are now relegated to corporate entities. The market metaphor conceals the inherent imperfections of the market and ignores the public nature of many aspects of medicine. This perspective also ignores the inability of the market to distribute goods and services whose supply and demand are unrelated to price. The metaphor pretends that there is such a thing as a free market in health insurance plans and that purchasers can and should be content with their choices when unexpected injuries or illnesses strike them or their family members. The reality is that American markets are highly regulated, major industries enjoy large public subsidies, industrial organizations tend toward oligopoly, and strong laws that protect consumers and offer them recourse through product-liability suits have become essential to prevent profits from being too ruthlessly pursued.

THE CLINTONS' MIXED METAPHORS

This summary of American medicine's two predominant metaphors helps explain why President Bill Clinton and Hillary Rodham Clinton were never able to articulate a coherent view of their goals for a reformed health care financing system. Their plan, according to the Clintons, rested on six pillars (or was guided by six "shining stars"): security, savings, choice, simplicity, responsibility, and quality. These six characteristics mix the military and market metaphors in impossible and inconsistent ways, and also introduce new, unrelated concepts..

The predominant metaphor of the Clintons seems to have been the military one: security was the first goal ("health care that will always be there"). But in the post-Cold War era, the pursuit of security as a reason to make a major change has been a tough sell. Even harder to sell was the idea of health care alliances as the centerpiece of the new security arrangement. The military metaphor (undercut by such words as "savings" and "choice") simply could not provide a coherent vision of the Clinton plan.

Nor could the market metaphor. The key concept of the market is, of course, consumer choice, and this was promised by the Clinton plan. The plan was founded on the choice of a health care plan, however, not on the choice of a physician or treatment. When the latter choices were seen as central (by television's Harry and Louise, for example, who said of government health care, "They choose, we lose"), the plan itself collapsed, and the alliances with it. Choice, quality and even savings can be generated by a market plan, but such an approach has little room for either responsibility or simplicity. In retrospect, the Clinton plan seems to have been doomed from the day its six inconsistent principles, goals or guidelines were articulated.

The Clintons also failed to engage the four negative characteristics of American culture that dominate medical care. Especially noteworthy is our denial of death. In perhaps the best response to the successful Harry-and-Louise campaign against their proposal, the Clintons taped a parody for the annual Gridiron Dinner. The centerpiece was the following dialogue:

> Hillary: On Page 12,743 . . . no, I got that wrong. It's Page 27,655; it says that eventually we are all going to die.
>
> Bill: Under the Clinton Health Plan? (*Hillary nods gravely*), You mean that after Bill and Hillary put all those new bureaucrats and taxes on us, we're still going to die?
>
> Hillary: Even Leon Panetta.
>
> Bill: Wow, that *is* scary! I've never been so frightened in all my life!
>
> Hillary: Me neither, Harry. (*They face the camera*)
>
> Bill and Hillary: There's *got* to be a better way.[10]

Some commentators, like ABC's Sam Donaldson, reacted by stating that one cannot discuss death in political discourse and have it help one's cause. The Clintons apparently agreed, and the White House refused to release copies of the videotape of the spoof even for educational use (and even though it had been broadcast on national television), adopting another leaf from military metaphor by treating the videotape as if it were a top-secret document.

THE ECOLOGIC METAPHOR

It seems reasonable to conclude that if Congress is ever to make meaningful progress in reforming our fast-changing system for financing and delivering medical care, a new way must be found to think about health itself. This will require at least a new metaphoric framework that permits us to reenvision and thus to reconstruct the American medical care system. I suggest that the leading candidate for a new metaphor is ecology.

Ecologists use words such as "integrity," "balance," "natural," "limited (resources)," "quality (of life)," "diversity," "renewable," "sustainable," "responsibility (for future generations)," "community" and "conservation."[11] If applied to health care, the concepts embedded in these words and others common to the ecology movement could have a profound influence on the way the debate about reform is conducted and on plans for change that are seen as reasonable. The ecologic metaphor could, for example, help us confront and accept limits (both on expectations about the length of our lives and on the expenditure of resources we think reasonable to increase longevity), value nature and emphasize the quality of life. This metaphor could lead us to worry about our grandchildren and thus to plan for the long term, to favor sustainable technology over technology we cannot afford to provide to all who could benefit from it, to emphasize prevention and public health measures, and to debate the merits of rationing.

Use of the ecologic metaphor is not unprecedented in medicine. Two physician writers, for example, have used it extensively. Lewis Thomas often invoked this metaphor in his essays in the *Journal,* and his idea that the earth itself could best be thought of as a "single cell" became the title for his first collection of essays, *The Lives of a Cell.*[12] Using this metaphor helped him, I think, to develop many of his important insights into modern medicine, including his concept of a "halfway technology," his argument that death should not be seen as the enemy, and his suggestion that in viewing humans as part of the environment, we could see ourselves from a new perspective, as highly specialized "handymen" for the earth.[12]

The other leading physician spokesperson for an ecologic view of medicine is Van Rensselaer Potter, who in coining the term "bioethics" in 1971 meant it to apply not just to medical ethics (its contemporary application) but to a blend of biologic knowledge and human values that would take special account of environmental values.[13] In his words, "Today we need biologists who respect the fragile web of life and who can broaden their knowledge to include the nature of man and his relation to the biological and physical worlds."[13]

Drawing on the attempts of the "deep ecologists" to ask more fundamental questions than their "shallow" environmental counterparts (who concentrate on the abatement of pollution and recycling),[14] psychiatrist Willard Gaylin fruitfully pointed out that the Clinton approach to health care reform was itself shallow.[15] He suggested – correctly, I think – that what was needed was a "wide-open far-ranging public debate about the deeper issues of health care – our attitudes toward life and death, the goals of medicine, the meaning of health, suffering versus survival, who shall live and who shall die (and who shall decide)."[15] Without addressing these deeper questions, Gaylin rightly argues, we can never solve our health care crisis.

The ecologic metaphor also naturally leads us to considerations of population health. This perspective shifts the emphasis from individual risk factors, for example, "toward the social structures and processes within which ill-health originates, and which will often be more amenable to modification."[16] Use of the ecologic metaphor encourages us to look upstream to see what is causing the illnesses and injuries downstream.[17] This is a reference to another metaphor, about villagers who devised complex methods to save people from drowning, instead of looking upstream to see who was pushing them in. The ecologic perspective puts more emphasis on prevention and public health interventions and less on wasteful interventions at the end of life.[18]

CONTROL AND COMMUNITY

The predominance of the military and market metaphors in our thinking about medicine has reinforced the quest for control that seems to define both modern medicine and postmodern politics. Medicine's accomplishments have been astonishing at both borders of life. Medical technology has, for example, eliminated the necessity to engage in sexual intercourse to procreate, and has thereby radically altered the meaning of parenthood in ways we have yet to confront socially. At life's other border, we continue our effort to banish death and, if unsuccessful, to assert control in the name of freedom to end life itself.

Unlike the military and market metaphors, which only reinforce our counterproductive American characteristics of wastefulness, obsession with technology, fear of death and individualism, the ecologic metaphor can help us confront them. Applied to medicine, the ecologic metaphor can encourage an alternative vision of resource conservation, sustainable technology, acceptance of death as natural and necessary, responsibility for others, and at least some degree of community.[19] It can also help move us from standards of medical practice determined by the law, an integral part of the market, to standards that provide a greater role for ethics and ethical behavior in the practice of medicine.

CONCLUSIONS

The challenge remains to create a health care system that provides affordable, high-quality care for all, and we will not face, let alone meet, this challenge if we continue to rely on visions of health care mediated by the military and market metaphors. Language has a powerful effect on how we think, and is infectious; as William S. Burroughs has aptly put it, "Language is a virus." We need a new vision of health care, and the ecologic metaphor provides one that can directly address the major problems with our current culture, as well as the deeper issues in health care. Physicians can invigorate the stagnant and depressing debate on health care reform by adopting a new metaphor that can in turn lead us to think and act in a new and productive way.

KEY IDEAS IN THIS ARTICLE:

- We have a health care system shaped by several primal and pervasive American values and characteristics; it is "wasteful, technologically driven, individualistic and death denying."

- In order to change this system in a meaningful way, we will have to "look deeper than money and means, to goals and ends – to devise a new metaphor to frame our discussion of public policy and to help us develop a new conception of health care."

- The military metaphor has had a pervasive influence on both the practice and financing of medicine in the United States.

- The military metaphor leads us to overmobilize, to ignore costs, to engage in medical arms races, to accept organizations that are hierarchical and dominated by men, to view the patient's body as a battlefield, to accept short-term, single-minded tactical goals, to concentrate on the physical, to see control as central, and to encourage expenditures of massive resources to achieve dominance.

- The market metaphor has decisively entered the health care culture. This metaphor emphasizes efficiency, profit maximization, customer satisfaction, the ability to pay, planning, entrepreneurship, and competition. Trust is replaced by "buyer beware," and there is no place for the poor and uninsured in the metaphor of the market.

- Nonprofit medical organizations tend to be corrupted by adopting the values of their for-profit competitors.

- Both the military and market metaphors *narrow* our vision, and neither can take us where we need to go. "I suggest that the leading candidate for a new metaphor is ecology."

- Central ideas of ecology – limited resources, quality of life, sustainable, community, conservation – could have a profound influence on the way the debate about reform is conducted and on plans for change.

- "The ecological metaphor could help us confront and accept limits, value nature, and emphasize the quality of life . . . lead us to worry about our grandchildren and thus to plan for the long term, to favor a sustainable technology over technology we cannot afford . . . to emphasize prevention and public health measures, and to debate the merits of rationing."

- "The ecological metaphor . . . leads us to considerations of population health. . . . shifts the emphasis toward the social structures and processes within which ill health originates, and which will often be more amenable to modification . . . encourages us to look upstream to see what is causing the illnesses and injuries downstream."

- "Applied to medicine, the ecological metaphor can encourage an alternative vision of resource conservation, sustainable technology, acceptance of death as natural and necessary, responsibility for others, and at least some degree of community.

A SUGGESTED PROCESS FOR REFLECTING ON THIS ARTICLE:

(See pages 234-254 for other processes that might better fit your specific goals and objectives.)

1. We have a health care system shaped by several primal and pervasive American values and characteristics; it is "wasteful, technologically driven, individualistic and death denying."

   In my family/religious/ethnic tradition, this echoes/conflicts with . . .

2. In order to change this system in a meaningful way, we will have to "look deeper than money and means, to goals and ends – to devise a new metaphor to frame our discussion of public policy and to help us develop a new conception of health care."

   In my family/religious/ethnic tradition, this echoes/conflicts with . . .

3. The market metaphor has decisively entered the health care culture. This metaphor emphasizes efficiency, profit maximization, customer satisfaction, the ability to pay, planning, entrepreneurship, and competition. Trust is replaced by "buyer beware," and there is no place for the poor and uninsured in the metaphor of the market.

   In my family/religious/ethnic tradition, this echoes/conflicts with . . .

4. Both the military and market metaphors *narrow* our vision, and neither can take us where we need to go.

   "I suggest that the leading candidate for a new metaphor is ecology."

   In my family/religious/ethnic tradition, this echoes/conflicts with . . .

5. "The ecological metaphor could help us confront and accept limits, value nature, and emphasize the quality of life . . . lead us to worry about our grandchildren and thus to plan for the long term, to favor a sustainable technology over technology we cannot afford . . . to emphasize prevention and public health measures, and to debate the merits of rationing."

   In my family/religious/ethnic tradition, this echoes/conflicts with . . .

6. "The ecological metaphor . . . leads us to considerations of population health . . . shifts the emphasis toward the social structures and processes within which ill health originates, and which will often be more amenable to modification . . . encourages us to look upstream to see what is causing the illnesses and injuries downstream."

   In my family/religious/ethnic tradition, this echoes/conflicts with . . .

7. "Applied to medicine, the ecological metaphor can encourage an alternative vision of resource conservation, sustainable technology, acceptance of death as natural and necessary, responsibility for others, and at least some degree of community.

   In my family/religious/ethnic tradition, this echoes/conflicts with . . .

8. In light of our discussion:

   - as (executive committee, as ethics committee, etc.), what are some next steps that we should take?

- as (hospital, home health agency, etc.), what are some next steps that we should take?

- what systems and structures call for special attention in order to improve the situation?

ENDNOTES

1. Lakoff G, Johnson M. Metaphors we live by. Chicago: University of Chicago Press, 1980.

2. Paternalism in health care. In: Childress JF. Who should decide? Paternalism in health care. New York: Oxford University Press, 1982:7.

3. Sontag S. Illness as metaphor and AIDS and its metaphors. New York: Doubleday, 1990.

4. Fussell P. The Great War and modern memory. New York: Oxford University Press, 1975.

5. Keegan J. A history of warfare. New York: Vintage Books, 1994:56-7.

6. Beisecker AE, Beisecker TD. Using metaphors to characterize doctor-patient relationships: paternalism versus consumerism. Health Commun 1993;5:41-58.

7. Eckholm E. While Congress remains silent, health care transforms itself. *New York Times.* December 18, 1994:1, 34.

8. Relman AS. The health care industry: where is it taking us? *N Engl J Med* 1991;325:854-9.

9. *Idem.* What market values are doing to medicine. *Atlantic Monthly.* March 1992:99-106.

10. Bill and Hill, auditions for "America's funniest health videos." *Boston Globe.* March 27, 1994:70.

11. Horwitz WA. Characteristics of environmental ethics: environmental activists' accounts. *Ethics Behav* 1994;4:345-67.

12. Thomas L. The lives of a cell. New York: Viking, 1974.

13. Potter VR. Bioethics: bridge to the future. Englewood Cliffs, N.J.: Prentice-Hall, 1971.

14. Sessions G, ed. Deep ecology for the twenty-first century. Boston: Shambhala, 1995.

15. Gaylin W. Faulty diagnosis: why Clinton's health-care plan won't cure what ails us. Harper's. October 1993:57-62.

16. Population health looking upstream. Lancet 1994;343:429-30.

17. McKinlay JB. A case for refocusing upstream: the political economy of illness. In: Proceedings of American Heart Association Conferences on Applying Behavioral Science to Cardiovascular Risk. Seattle: American Health Association, 1974:7-17.

18. Dubos R. Mirage of health. New York: Harper, 1959:233.

19. Friedman E. An ethic for all of us. *Healthcare Forum J* 1991;34:11-3.

PART 2

READINGS IN INSTITUTIONAL
ETHICS OF MANAGED CARE

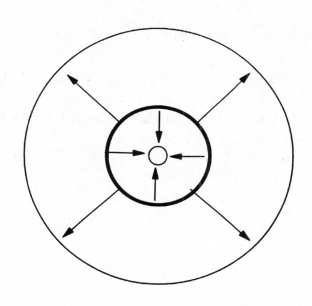

The articles in this section help us think about some select questions of how institutions should understand and manage health care. While many immediate possibilities of MCO behavior are substantially shaped and limited by decisions and definitions on the societal level, the MCO still has significant areas of freedom and influence for which it is responsible. What is a good and virtuous MCO? What are the systems and structures that an MCO should have in place to meet its multiple duties to its own mission, the society of which it is part and the individuals that make it up as patients and staff?

The literature contained in this section tends to emphasize duties to individuals, and primarily to members. This is historically understandable and to a great extent appropriate. One can compensate for deficiencies in this regard by moving discussions and explorations in desired directions through the formats used for group interaction.

CHAPTER 7

MANAGED CARE: JEKYLL OR HYDE?

Carolyn M. Clancy, MD, Howard Brody, MD, PhD

THE TOPIC MOST DISCUSSED BY PHYSICIANS TODAY IS THE INCREASING percentage of US health care being taken over by managed care organizations.[1] While physicians in practice are struggling to interpret the requirements and implications of contracts with emerging or established health care systems,[2] many academic medical centers have also joined the "dance of vertical integration."[3,4] What has not emerged from the offtimes emotional discussions is a cogent examination of the impact of the transformation of medical practice from a cottage industry to a corporate enterprise on how we deliver care, assess and improve the quality of care, and educate future physicians. It is an urgent matter, then, for the medical profession to address the ethical principles that will preserve a sound physician-patient relationship within this rapidly changing environment.

To address the ethics of the physician-patient relationship in managed care realistically and insightfully, we must keep several issues in mind. To avoid any temptation to confuse ethics with either habit or financial self-interest, we must recognize that no system of reimbursement is devoid of financial self-interest. Fee-for-service encourages doing more rather than less; capitation may encourage the reverse. The increasing scrutiny of the costs of clinical decisions and the subsequent transfer of care from individual practitioners to large organizations has radically torqued the framework for ethical decision-making. Physicians cannot ignore that decisions related to resource allocation are, in fact, being made, but must strive to ensure that those decisions do not adversely impact the health of patients. While managed care makes trade-offs between individual patients more explicit, this does not mean that those trade-offs were not always present, however implicitly.[5] Finally, we must recognize the diversity of organizations currently included in the broad category of "managed care," and avoid ethical dicta that treat all of those settings as identical.

We agree with Emanuel et al[6] that managed care can, in some instances, enhance the ethical quality of the physician-patient relationship, even as it threatens it in other ways.[7] We believe, however, that we can go farther in identifying features of managed care organizations that improve rather than threaten the physician-patient relationship. Current technology is inadequate because it does not facilitate understanding of the commonalities or differences in the managed care industry alphabet soup of labels (HMO,

PPO, PHO, IPA, EPO, POS, and so on) and the potential for promoting ethical physician-patient relationships. Lacking suitable alternatives, we propose "Jekyll care" and "Hyde care."

JEKYLL CARE

The Jekyll plan encourages personal and long-standing relationships between the patient and the primary provider, a commitment to caring for the same population of patients over time, and a population-based approach to medical practice that incorporates public health as well as individual medical care strategies. The plan cannot work unless it creates a culture of practice characterized by practitioners who equate good patient care with cost-effective care, carefully measures outcomes to identify quality problems and strategies for improvement, and values collaborative relationships between primary care physicians and subspecialists to define the optimal mix of interventions for each patient. Jekyll plans are more frequently found among the older staff model health maintenance organizations that were established in the 1940s through the 1960s, when cost containment was an unexpected benefit rather than the central purpose. The management structure guarantees that bottom-line fiscal considerations do not intrude unduly on the medical decisions that providers make on behalf of individual patients. Put simply, the management structure harasses physicians who routinely prescribe a $60 bottle of antihistamines when the patient would get just as much improvement with a $6 bottle, but does not harass physicians who have sicker patients and appropriately provide more intensive levels of care for them.[8] Profits are invested in improvements in patient care.

HYDE CARE

This model is more commonly found among the newest generation of managed care organizations, often begun by insurers who have no previous experience in providing care, to corner market share by offering local employers a "managed care product." The plan assembles a nominal network of primary care providers, subspecialists, hospitals, home care agencies, and other components. Lacking a significant clinical leadership structure to create the "culture of practice" that characterizes Jekyll plans, Hyde plans can only control costs by alternative means – exclusion of sicker patients, rationing by inconvenience, burdensome micromanagement of clinical decisions, or denial of beneficial but expensive care to some patients, either by micromanagement or by perverse incentives for providers. Because no real teamwork develops among providers of different specialties, primary and specialty physicians often feel themselves pitted against each other as the plan strives to ratchet down costs.[9] Profits are returned to stockholders.

The American Medical Association Council on Ethical and Judicial Affairs report, "Ethical Issues in Managed Care,"[10] offers much sound advice, but it fails to come to terms with two basic issues: the inherent tension between calling for individual patients and populations of patients, and the physician's role in resource allocation. One section of the report, "Conflicts

Among Patients," examines some allocation decisions, but fails to articulate a basic truth recently stated by Eddy[11]: "When physicians hoard resources for their own patients, they are not taking from administrators or insurers; they are taking from other patients." The report assumes that harm inevitably results when the physician withholds a potentially beneficial, even if costly, treatment from the individual patient. There is no explicit acknowledgment that so long as resources are finite, the physician who devotes expensive and marginally beneficial resources to the care of patient A, might through that act be harming patients X, Y, and Z, who could have benefited much more substantially had those same resources been made available elsewhere. The physician's assumption that A is "my" patient, while X, Y, and Z are "someone else's," needs to be confronted as a basic question of social justice. The assumption is not credible in Jekyll care; in a Hyde care system, distinguishing other patients' needs from those of stockholders is problematic.

A related lack of clarity exists in the report's condemnation of "bedside rationing" without specifying what is being condemned. How should ethical managed care organizations allocate resources? Cassel[12] has proposed criteria for physicians' ethical involvement in resource allocation: universal access to a basic minimum level of care, physicians' levels of income must not be directly related to treatment choices, a closed financial system within which meaningful trade-offs can be made, and an ethically acceptable framework for decision-making. Failure of national legislation to guarantee universal coverage leaves physicians with a less-than-optimum framework for ethical considerations, but refusing to confront reality may harm patients. The fairest and most defensible principle would be to try to match treatments with those patients most likely to benefit, and to begin to discourage or to withhold expensive treatments when patients whose chance of benefiting is very slim or nearly zero can be identified. This process can be applied by faceless bureaucrats consulting computer protocols; appropriately, the Council recognizes that procedures will be much finer-tuned, and more equitably distributed, when physicians take into account the nuances of individual patients' medical histories and conditions.[12]

Still, the Council's recommendations in this regard invite clarification. The report states that physicians routinely make judgments about costs and benefits, that physicians should ensure that resource allocation is guided by medically relevant information, that it is unethical to waste resources, and that physicians have a duty to advocate for an individual patient's right to treatment that might be materially beneficial. Should the reader conclude that physicians should sit at the patient's bedside and decide not to administer certain treatments because they would be wasteful, or decide that, because of certain peculiarities, this patient has so great a chance of benefiting that a certain treatment ought to be used, even if some guideline proscribes the treatment? What if the same physician, using the same process of reasoning, decides that this patient has so low a chance of benefiting that the resources could better be used elsewhere (i.e., agreeing that predetermined guidelines do apply in this particular case)? Has that physician now crossed over into an ethical no-fly zone?

We believe more guidance is needed, and that it would be much more useful to admit that some sort of bedside rationing is inevitable unless we are to have totally bureaucratic and depersonalized decision-making. The ethical imperative is to specify how to make these decisions responsibly. The Council's recommendations that decisions at a policy level be separated from those at a clinical level, and that managed care plans create structures similar to hospital medical staffs, are a good beginning. These recommendations must lead to a more extended dialogue among the profession that will encompass the many current dilemmas physicians encounter.

For example, in an extreme version of unethical practice, a Hyde plan might discourage physicians from meeting patients' needs adequately through perverse financial incentives to physicians, and then forbid the providers from informing patients about these limitations with a form of gag order written into their employment contract.[14,15] Full disclosure of incentives is barred if physicians' contracts forbid such disclosure. Individual practitioners may face a Hobson's choice to speak out, but the voice of the profession should be unambiguous against such gag rules. Similarly, Hyde plans may discourage dissemination of interventions that truly improve patient outcomes in the name of proprietary interests.[16] Both all-too-real scenarios directly conflict with long-standing professional traditions of complete disclosure and sharing advances with professional colleagues to ensure their broad dissemination. Reluctance or timidity of the profession to confront and resolve these conflicts will reduce physicians to technicians oblivious to long-standing ethical and professional traditions, and may result in reduced quality of care for patients.

As managed care systems assume a larger role in American health care, we urgently need to address the following questions: How do we increase the proportion of Jekyll plans? What can be done to transform Hyde plans into Jekyll plans? How can physicians in Jekyll plans work together most effectively to assess and improve quality of care? How do we train tomorrow's physicians in the Jekyll "culture of practice" so as to eliminate the need to retrain new physicians into a population-based approach to health care? The ultimate outcome of the current (revolution can only be positive if the profession insists on a leadership role to encourage the beneficial aspects of managed care, eliminate those features that counter patients' interests, and work toward a system focused on health outcomes rather than financial interests.

KEY IDEAS IN THIS ARTICLE:

- The emergence and rapid spread of managed care has raised concerns about the integrity of the physician-patient relationship.

- Some forms of managed care are more conducive to preserving the physician-patient relationship than others. Those that support the therapeutic relationship are referred to as "Jekyll care," and those that threaten it are called "Hyde care." They represent both ends of a spectrum.

- Jekyll managed care is perhaps best exemplified in the more traditional staff model HMOs established in the 1940s through the 1960s. The culture of practice in these plans is characterized by cost-effective care, efforts to improve quality, and collaboration between primary care physicians and subspecialists. Cost containment, while important, is not primary, and bottom-line concerns do not unduly intrude on treatment decisions for individual patients. Profits are reinvested in patient care. These plans take a population-based approach that combines preventive and acute care and fosters continuity of care, with both individual patients and its population of covered lives.

- Hyde care is represented by newer forms of managed care often begun by insurers with little or no clinical experience. Instead of Jekyll care's culture of practice, they attempt to control costs by excluding sicker patients from their plans, rationing by inconveniencing patients, micromanaging clinical decisions, and offering perverse incentives to providers. Collaboration between primary care physicians and subspecialists is usually absent. Cost containment and profits are central concerns, and profits are returned to stockholders.

A SUGGESTED PROCESS FOR REFLECTING ON THIS ARTICLE:

(See pages 234-254 for other processes that might better fit your specific goals and objectives.)

	Additional Characteristics	Characteristics in our Organization	Implications/Response
Jekyll Care			
Hyde Care			

Are there ways to increase "Jekyll characteristics" and to reduce "Hyde characteristics" in your own organization? What concrete steps would need to be taken? What obstacles might be encountered? What might be the consequences of such efforts?

ENDNOTES

1. Iglehart JF. The struggle between managed care and fee-for-service practice. *N Engl J Med.* 1994;331:63-67.

2. Williams BJ. The train is leaving the station. *N Engl J Med.* 1994;331:1316-1317.

3. Kassirer JP. Academic medical centers under siege. *N Engl J Med.* 1994;331: 1370-1371.

4. Iglehart JK. Rapid changes for academic medical centers. *N Engl J Med.* 1994;331:1391-1395.

5. Friedman E. Doctors and rationing: the end of the honor system. *Prim Care.* 1986;13:349-364.

6. Emanuel EJ, Mezey M, Dubler NN. Preserving the physician-patient relationship in the era of managed care. *JAMA* 1995;273:323-329.

7. Franks P, Clancy C, Nutting P. Gatekeeping revisited: protecting patients from overtreatment. *N Engl J Med.* 1992;327:424-429.

8. Yelin EH, Shearn MA, Epstein WV. Health outcomes for a chronic disease in prepaid group practice and fee-for-service settings: the case of rheumatoid arthritis. *Med Care.* 1986:24:236-247.

9. Roulides ZC, Schulman KA. Physician communication in managed care organizations: opinions of primary care physicians. J Fam Pract. 1994;39:446-451.

10. Council on Ethical and Judicial Affairs, American Medical Association. Ethical issues in managed care. *JAMA.* 1994;273:330-335

11. Eddy DM. Rationing resources while improving quality: how to get more for less. *JAMA.* 1994;272:817-824.

12. Cassel CK. Doctors and allocation decisions: a new role in the new Medicare. *J Health Polit Policy Law.* 1985;10:549-564.

13. Welch HG. Should the health care forest be selectively thinned by physicians or clear cut by payers? *Ann Intern Med.* 1991;115:223-226.

14. HMO physician payment: notes from the underground. *Phys Natl Health Program Newletter.* October 1994:3.

15. Passaro V. Better try not to get sick. *New York Times.* October 11, 1993:A11.

16. Berwick DB. Making clinical practice guidelines useful. Presented at the Agency for Health Care Policy and Research Conference; November 8, 1994; Rockville, Md.

CHAPTER 8

MEDICAL ETHICS IN THE ERA OF MANAGED CARE: THE NEED FOR INSTITUTIONAL STRUCTURES INSTEAD OF PRINCIPLES FOR INDIVIDUAL CASES

Ezekiel J. Emanuel

MEDICAL ETHICS MUST STOP BEING CASE-ORIENTED AND BECOME institutionally oriented. We bioethicists must stop approaching problems from a philosophical perspective and adopt a political science perspective. Nothing makes this more clear than the challenges of managed care.

Traditionally, medical ethics has focused on cases and the ethical issues that arise between individual physicians and patients. For instance, analysis of informed consent has focused on what the physician is obligated to disclose to his or her patient; cases regarding the termination of care have focused on decision-making for patients such as Karen Quinlan and Nancy Cruzan; and cases regarding confidentiality have focused on when it is proper to reveal specific information about patients. It is by adopting the philosophical approach and focusing on the principles and rules that should apply to such cases that medical ethics has been most successful. By contrast, medical ethics has not been as successful in addressing the influence of institutional arrangements in resolving these ethical issues and in problems that involve the healthcare system. This is probably most clear in the rather disappointing contribution medical ethics has made to the problem of allocating healthcare resources. While we have been able to delineate broad principles, these have had little practical significance for actual decisions regarding the allocation of resources. Similarly, we have been rather poor at elucidating the type of institutional arrangements that affect fulfillment of the requirements of informed consent or confidentiality in individual cases.

This focus on ethical principles and rules is no longer tenable – if it ever was. The advent and explosive growth of managed care has dramatically and irreversibly changed the nature of medical practice, and therefore the context in which medical ethical issues arise. The physician-patient interaction no longer occurs in a practitioner's office in which the practitioner, alone or in a small group of colleagues, has control over the structures that influence the interaction. Instead these interactions occur within large organizations in which the practitioner or a small group of colleagues does not control the "rules of engagement." The context of medical ethics can no longer be cases, but institutional structures.

I propose to consider what institutional structures we might adopt in the era of managed care to ensure that patients' welfare is protected.

MANAGED CARE'S THREAT TO THE WELFARE OF PATIENTS

The dramatic rise of managed care in the 1990s is a response to many problems within the American healthcare system, in particular, to uncontrolled costs. Managed care has two primary techniques to control costs: financial incentives and guidelines or protocols. In managed care, the financial incentives – primarily capitation, salary "withholds," and bonus arrangements – are meant to put the physician "at financial risks" for the care delivered to patients. In practice, this means physicians should lose money if they provide too many services to patients. It is hoped that by putting physicians "at risk" they will – individually or collectively – carefully determine necessary and valuable services and provide them, and concomitantly withhold services that are unnecessary or of marginal value to the patient. Advocates of putting physicians "at risk" maintain that it is the most effective – if not the only – way to ensure that physicians seriously evaluate services and do not provide those that are unnecessary or marginal. These advocates seem to believe what the Australian health minister is reported to have said at a 1994 Organization for Economic Cooperation and Development conference: "If you want to be sure that physicians get the message, be sure you write it on a check."[1]

The obvious ethical problem with putting physicians "at risk" is that it creates a conflict of interest. Lee Goldman and I have distinguished two types of conflicts of interest: conflicts of commission, in which there are financial incentives to provide more services, which is inherent in the fee-for-service reimbursement system; and conflicts of omission, in which there are financial incentives to provide fewer services, which is inherent in the capitation reimbursement system.[2] The ethical evaluation of both conflicts of interest is clear: they are wrong because they have the tendency to make the physician's personal interest supersede what should be the primary interest: the health of the patient. Just as we have devised mechanisms to limit conflicts of commission, we also have to devise mechanisms to limit conflicts of omission.

Guidelines or protocols can serve many purposes. One is to standardize care. However, in devising guidelines, there are inadequate data to clearly determine what constitutes the optimal approach to the care of patients. Similarly, even where there are substantial data, the data might conflict. In such situations, there will be a judgment call about what services to include and what services to exclude. Such judgments can be affected by financial interests. In addition, there may be certain services that are clearly beneficial, but of substantial cost, and other services that are less than optimal, but save significant resources. Decisions about whether to include these services or not will also be judgment calls that can be influenced by financial incentives. Frequently the conflicts of interest that arise in devising guidelines affect administrators of managed-care plans.

Current reports suggest that financial incentives and guidelines are widely used in managed care. According to the Physician Payment Review Commission study released in 1995, almost all of the managed-care plans used financial incentives, and the majority of them thought it was the single most effective technique to control costs.[3] Similarly, almost two-thirds of managed-care plans used guidelines, and 80% assessed whether physicians complied with these guidelines.[4] There is a paucity of data about how these financial incentives and guidelines affect the care of patients. The only study we have is from Hillman in 1989, in which he found that the use of financial incentives was associated with fewer hospital days, fewer patient visits, and the profitability of managed-care plans.[5] We have no direct data on whether these financial conflicts or guidelines actually result in adverse outcomes for patients. We might wait to devise rules for these conflicts of omission that arise from these mechanisms until we have more definitive data regarding their adverse effects on the care of patients. Instead I suggest that we act prophylactically. One of the main reasons is to reassure the public. There is widespread suspicion that conflicts of omission in managed care will lead to worse care for patients and their families. The only way to regain the confidence of patients and the general public is to create institutional structures that minimize these conflicts or, putting it another way, to create incentives that counterbalance the financial incentives.

INSTITUTIONAL STRUCTURES TO MINIMIZE CONFLICTS OF OMISSION

Lee Goldman and I have suggested six structures that could counter conflicts of omission: (1) professionalism, (2) disclosure, (3) competition, (4) prospective review of financial incentives, (5) prospective review of guidelines, and (6) mediation and appeals procedures.[6] Here I can only briefly comment on the first four.

PROFESSIONALISM

By professionalism, I mean the rededication of physicians to the professional ideal that the welfare of patients is the physician's primary goal, which should not be superseded by a physician's personal financial interest. Kassirer has recently suggested that professionalism is the primary mechanism that should be adopted to counter conflicts of omission.[7]

Professionalism is important, and therefore is a necessary protection of the welfare of patients. However, it is not sufficient for two reasons. First, as we have learned from the data that has accumulated on conflicts of commission, it is not a sufficiently robust value and incentive to ensure the protection of patients. Some physicians – probably a small minority, but still an important group – are willing to subvert patients' welfare for their own financial gain, and even try to rationalize this. There is no reason to think that the tendency to have conflicts of omission that endanger patients' welfare will be less under managed care.

Second, professionalism harkens back to the old medical ethics that focuses on principles and rules for cases, that adopts the philosophical perspective and fails to appreciate the necessity of focusing on the need to create institutional structures that more systematically foster ethical behavior and protect the welfare of patients.

DISCLOSURE

The traditional response to a conflict of interest by ethicists is disclosure. Physicians – and others – who have a conflict or potential conflict should reveal it and let the patient act on the information. This is the approach adopted by many medical schools, by journals, and recommended in the *Moore* ruling.[8]

Again, while disclosure is necessary, it is by no means sufficient. First, it is not "holy water" that purifies unethical acts and behavior. Some financial incentives and use of guidelines may be unethical – even if not illegal – and disclosure does not magically make them acceptable. Furthermore, disclosure works only when the person who is informed can change his or her behavior in response to the information. In a competitive healthcare marketplace, it is likely that managed-care plans will have similar, if not identical, financial incentives and guidelines. This is likely to preclude patients from acting on the disclosed information.

COMPETITION

Under some scenarios of the development of managed care, price competition stops because all managed-care plans reduce hospitalization and numbers of physicians, and provide services at similar prices. Once this has occurred – and according to some commentators it is happening in the most mature managed-care markets in California – competition turns to ensuring the quality of services. In this scenario, managed-care plans monitor quality, and thereby ensure financial incentives and guidelines do not threaten the welfare of patients.

This is not the place to discuss the probability of this scenario. Even its proponents acknowledge important limitations to competition as a mechanism of ensuring quality. Probably the major limitation involves the science and capability of quality assessment, which is in its infancy. The Healthplan Employer Data Information Sheet (HEDIS), for instance, contains only nine quality measures, with the focus on screening tests. The limited number of services it assesses encourages "gaming" the system. Managed-care plans might focus on the assessed service, yet ignore those services that are unassessed. For instance, there is a heavy emphasis on the percentage of eligible patients receiving mammography in these quality-assessment scans. One problem with this is that it says nothing about the quality of care received by patients who have breast cancer; a high proportion of women can be screened – which is good – but we also need to be sure those with cancer receive good care. In addition, many quality measures focus on medical services with short-term outcomes, such as 30-day mortality from surgical procedures or myocardial infarctions, rather than treatment of diseases with long-term outcomes.

Further, we lack the risk adjustments that are necessary to conduct quality assessments across many different providers.

Thus, whatever the likelihood that competition can ensure patients' welfare, it depends on the advancement of quality assessment. At the moment, quality assessment is not sufficiently developed for us to place much confidence in it, and it is uncertain when it will be fully developed to ensure high-quality care for patients. Again, while competition might be helpful, it is not a sufficient protection for patients.

REVIEW OF FINANCIAL INCENTIVES

Financial incentives for physicians to limit services that may be beneficial to patients – either through capitation, salary withholds or bonuses for reduced use of services – is a primary threat to the welfare of patients. In general, we should encourage financial incentives that (1) are spread over the performance of many physicians, such as the physicians in a managed-care site or region, and (2) focus on substantial health outcomes, not specialty referrals or the utilization of services. Furthermore, we should establish principles that set limits for the total use of financial incentives. In particular, in the area of conflicts of commission, we have a principle that the higher the financial incentive, the larger the conflict; at some point, the financial incentive is simply too large and so must be prohibited. For conflicts of omission, when the salary withhold or bonus exceeds 20% of a physician's salary, it is too large, and should be prohibited.

Applying these general rules to the specific contracts between managed-care plans and physicians may be difficult. In some cases, the rules may be too restrictive; in other cases, the influence of other incentives may have to be considered. Thus, I suggest that there should be prospective review of all financial incentives by an independent board. This board should include not just physicians and management, but other interested and objective parties, including patients' representatives, ethicists, lawyers, and possibly government officials. Indeed, there is some move by the New Jersey and North Carolina state medical licensing boards to review financial incentives in physicians' contracts. While a licensing board may not be the proper forum, it does suggest many people are coming to see the merits of such a review process.

CONCLUSION

Managed care has fundamentally changed the nature of medical ethical issues. They no longer arise in the context of individual patients and physicians. Instead they arise in the context of complex institutions that establish an organizational framework in which these ethical issues arise. To address medical ethical issues, we must change our focus from articulating principles and rules that apply to individual cases to devising institutional structures that can ensure ethical behavior. This article briefly reviews some of the proposals that Dr. Goldman and I have made about the kinds of institutional structures that should be considered in protecting the patient's welfare from conflicts of interest of omission. These institutional structures are not meant to be exhaustive, but simply to begin medical ethicists thinking about how to address ethical problems in a new way.

KEY IDEAS IN THIS ARTICLE:

- The explosive growth of managed care has dramatically and irreversibly changed the nature of medical practice and, hence, the context in which medical ethical issues arise.

- Given this new context, a primary focus on the physician-patient relationship or on cases is no longer adequate.

- Nor are the traditional principles of medical ethics adequate.

- Rather, medical ethicists, if they are to have anything to say to managed care, must adopt an institutional, political science perspective instead of the usual case-based, clinical and philosophical approach and focus.

- The conflict of interest for physicians that results from financial incentives is a good example. The only way to address this problem is to create institutional structures to minimize the conflict. One might consider four possible "structural changes": a rededication of physicians to the primacy of patient welfare; disclosure of conflicts of interest to patients; an emphasis on quality; alterations in the way financial incentives are structured. While the first three are necessary, they are not sufficient. Only the last involves a change in structure that might have a more lasting effect.

A SUGGESTED PROCESS FOR REFLECTING ON THIS ARTICLE:

(See pages 234-254 for other processes that might better fit your specific goals and objectives.)

1. Imagine that you are a member of an organizational ethics committee. Identify some aspect of managed care in your institution that you believe to be ethically problematic. Bring it before the larger committee for discussion. In your discussion, consider the following:

Morally Problematic Aspect of Managed Care	Reasons Why It Is Morally Problematic	Positive & Negative Consequences of this Aspect	Alternative Structure(s)	Obstacles & Next Steps

2. Does your institution have mechanisms in place for addressing ethical issues in managed care? If yes, what are they? Do they work well? Why? Why not?

If no, why is this the case? What might be done to alter this situation? What challenges would need to be addressed for this to occur?

ENDNOTES

1. Organization for Economic Development conference, Australia, 1994.

2. E.J. Emanuel and L. Goldman, "Protecting Patient Welfare in Managed Care: The Need for Collective Action," (manuscript).

3. Physician Payment Review Commission, *Arrangements Between Managed Care Plans and Physicians* (Washington, D.C.: PPRC, February 1995).

4. *Ibid.*

5. A.L. Hillman, M.V. Pauly, and J.J. Kerstein, "How Do Financial Incentives Affect Physicians' Clinical Decisions and the Financial Performance of Health Maintenance Organizations?" *New England Journal of Medicine* 321 (1989): 86-92.

6. Emanuel and Goldman, see note 2 above.

7. J.P. Kassirer, "Managed Care and the Morality of the Marketplace," *New England Journal of Medicine* 330 (1995): 50-52.

8. *Moore v. Regents of the University of California* 271, Cal Rptr. 146 (1990).

CHAPTER 9

BUSINESS VS. MEDICAL ETHICS: CONFLICTING STANDARDS FOR MANAGED CARE

Wendy K. Mariner

THE INCREASED COMPETITION FOR A SHARE OF THE MARKET OF INSURED patients, which arose in the wake of failed comprehensive health care reform, has provoked questions about what, if any, standards will govern new "competitive" health care organizations.[1] Managed care arrangements, which typically shift to providers and patients some or all of the financial risk for patient care,[2] are of special concern because they can create incentives to withhold beneficial care from patients.[3] Of course, fee-for-service (FFS) medical practice creates incentives to provide unnecessary services, and managed care can avoid that type of harm.[4] Still, as Edmund Pellegrino has noted, "managed care, by its nature, places the good of the patient into conflict with . . . (1) the good of all the other patients served by the plan; (2) the good of the plan and the organization, themselves . . . ; and (3) the self-interest of the physician."[5]

These potential conflicts have sparked a small flurry of articles and conferences that examine the "ethics" of managed care.[6] Participants in this discussion recognize the benefits of managed care, including its focus on disease prevention and health promotion (long overdue in American medical practice), its coordination of services based on the totality of a patient's health needs (rather than on isolated responses to specific symptoms), and its ability to hold down premiums. Yet financial incentives to limit services may undermine managed care's ability to achieve such benefits.

Carolyn Clancy and Howard Brody distinguish good managed care organizations (MCOs), which they call "Jekyll care" from "bad" organizations or "Hyde care."[7] In their view, Jekyll organizations typically are well-established, nonprofit health maintenance organizations (HMOs), like Group Health Cooperative of Puget Sound and Kaiser-Permanente Foundation, that encourage coordinated care, including preventive services, in long-term personal relationships between patients and primary care providers. They find bad managed care most often in the newer, investor-owned, for-profit entities operated by insurance companies and managers.[8] With little or no experience in health care delivery, such organizations may focus on cutting costs and on ensuring an adequate return on investment to their shareholders.

The idea that some managed care is good and some bad suggests that some socially accepted standard can be defined against which to judge individual plans. But, we have no such standard yet. Indeed, disagreement persists over whether any standard is even necessary. Among those who advocate particular standards, there is implicit disagreement on whether the standard should be based on principles of economics, policy, or ethics; and if ethical principles apply, whether they should be medical ethics or business ethics.

This article explores the difficulty of adopting ethical standards for MCOs. First, it is not clear what counts as an ethical standard for an organization. The ideals of quality and efficiency are desirable goals, but do not describe how they ought to be achieved. The ethical principles that promote free and fair competition are quite different from the ethical principles that preserve the integrity of the physician-patient relationship, and specifically those that protect patient welfare, and these principles can lead to quite different outcomes. MCOs were created to achieve economic objectives that may be fundamentally incompatible with traditional principles of medical ethics. Moreover, in today's open-ended health care system, it is questionable whether American economic institutions are susceptible to purely moral suasion. Thus, even if it is possible to agree that certain ethical principles ought to apply to managed care, the market may make it impossible to live fully by those principles.

Finally, it is important not to mistake ethical managed care for an ethical national health care system. Good MCOs may be able to provide efficient, high-quality care; but, in the long run, they are not likely to be able to do so and simultaneously cut costs and promote equitable access to care. If the analysis presented here is correct, then we have a choice: either abandon the goal of universal access to health care, or regulate the health care system by eliminating those marketplace standards that conflict with equitable access to care.

ECONOMIC AND POLITICAL GOALS FOR MANAGED CARE

Ethical principles are sometimes conflated with economic and political goals. When the Clinton administration's task force was developing the Health Security Act, it invited a group of ethicists to propose principles for the plan. The group's list of 14 principles was reduced to the following six for presentation to the public: security, savings, choice, quality, responsibility and simplicity.[9] These may be laudable goals for health care reform, but with the possible exception of choice and responsibility, they are not ethical principles.

The current growth of MCOs is encouraged as an alternative to comprehensive health care reform.[10] The Clinton administration's proposal provoked successful opposition from groups who argued that additional government intervention was not needed in the health insurance market because increased competition could achieve the goals of controlling costs and providing good quality care.[11] (They did not claim that competition could achieve universal access to care.) Were care "managed" properly, it could maintain quality and lower costs (or at least limit cost increases). Thus, the goals of managed care came to be seen as the efficient use of health care resources (or controlling costs) to provide quality care.[12] The most politically appealing argument was cost-control; and managed care is advocated first and foremost as a cost-control mechanism by those who oppose additional government intervention in health care financing.[13]

Today, health insurers only have a limited number of ways to save money: use resources efficiently; pay providers less; shift the risk of loss to providers; exclude costly patients from coverage; reduce covered benefits; limit services and deny treatment claims; and increase deductibles and copayments. It is certainly possible to increase efficiency, and avoid waste and duplication of services, in administering and delivering health care.[14] Still, many knowledgeable commentators believe that, in the long run, efficiency alone will not reduce costs enough to avoid limiting the amount of beneficial services needed by patients,[15] especially where the patient population includes an increasing number of older, sicker people.

The remaining cost-control methods are likely to result in reducing services available to patients or increasing patients' out-of-pocket expenditures. For example, insurers can reduce their own costs by lowering the amount they pay providers – especially hospitals and physicians – to care for patients, either by obtaining fee discounts, or by paying providers on a capitated basis (a fixed fee per subscriber) in whole or in part, so that the provider bears the risk of financial loss if the costs of care exceed the capitation fee.[16] Managed care plans may use practice guidelines, quality control committees, and financial rewards and penalties to influence physicians' treatment decisions.[17] Plans may also require patient care to be screened by primary care gatekeepers, and employ or contract only with physicians who practice in a cost-saving manner and adhere to the plan's efficient treatment methods.

Historically, most insurers avoided large or unpredictable expenses by refusing to insure patients who were at risk of needing expensive services.[18] The practice of "cherrypicking," or insuring only healthy patients who are unlikely to get sick, is still an effective cost-control device.[19] Plans can also encourage patients who require expensive services to leave the plan and join another by, for example, providing poor or inconvenient service, refusing desired care, or not responding to complaints.[20]

Health plans can limit their expenses by reducing the number and type of medical benefits covered by the plan. Where services are not expressly excluded from the contract, insurers may deny coverage on the grounds that they are not medically necessary, for example.[21] Finally, increased deductibles and copayments shift to patients a larger proportion of the cost of their care, although their contribution to insurer cost savings may be minimal.

The goals of efficiency and quality care are desirable programmatic goals for health plans, but they do not specify ethical standards for their achievement. They may also conflict with one another. Efficiency is unlikely to control costs enough to avoid hard decisions about limitations on care. Defining and measuring quality of care remains problematic.[22] In such circumstances, ethical standards to guide MCOs' actions appear especially needed.

DIFFERENCES IN MEDICAL ETHICS AND BUSINESS ETHICS

Can and should ethical standards apply to MCOs? The answer to such a question depends on what counts as an ethical standard. Traditional principles of medical ethics that govern the physician-patient relationship certainly have a role to play in the delivery of medical care, whether it is done in private FFS practice or in integrated service networks.[23] MCOs, however, do more than deliver medical care. They combine insurance, management and care delivery. It may be argued that the organization itself does not deliver medical care; its physicians and nurses do. The organization is an economic entity, often a corporation – a legal fiction, not a person in a profession with a history of professional ethics. Thus, the ethical principles that have traditionally been thought to apply to health care practitioners do not easily fit MCOs.

Susan Wolf has rightly distinguished between physicians' ethics and organizational ethics, arguing for the development of ethical standards for health care organizations.[24] That task faces several obstacles. First, it is debatable whether organizations are moral entities or capable of having ethics at all.[25] Wolf argues that health care organizations qualify as moral agents because they "specify levels of management and care delivery, formulate rules and policies, and consider moral reasons." Of course most, if not all, organizations (including Microsoft and R.J. Reynolds) formulate rules and policies and consider moral reasons for their actions. The fact that corporations make decisions based on moral reasoning does not mean that they must. These two criteria alone do not suffice to describe an institutional moral agent.

What distinguishes health care organizations from other (commercial and nonprofit) enterprises is the fact that they are in the business of delivering health care (Wolf's first factor). Moreover, that health care is actually provided by individual professionals who do have ethical obligations. MCOs perform both medical and business functions, taking actions to provide or withhold care that touch the traditional sphere of medical ethics, and, at the same time, acting like ordinary business enterprises with no moral obligations or, at least, obligations that have little to do with traditional medical ethics. This functional duality gives health care organizations a foot in both the medical and the business camps.

However, it is not necessary to confer moral agency on organizations in order to hold them to ethical standards of conduct. Whether or not organizations are moral entities or have moral rights or duties, their actions can be judged by moral standards and either praised or condemned.[26] Organizations can voluntarily create institutional structures and policies that require or encourage ethical behavior on the part of their personnel. Moreover, ethical standards of conduct can be legally imposed where it is socially desirable to achieve important goals.[27] The more difficult tasks will be developing the content of standards that take into account the dual business and medical functions of MCOs, and ensuring that organizations can adhere to such standards in an increasingly competitive environment.

The types of standards that have been proposed for managed care entities tend to reflect different conceptions of the organization – either its medical functions or its business functions, but not both. Those who seek ethical standards to ensure the delivery of high quality care appear to conceive of the organization as an entity that has or should have moral obligations because of its medical care functions.[28] The standards they propose focus on preserving physicians' traditional (or updated) ethical commitment to patient welfare, despite financial and management controls designed to restrict the cost of care. Others appear to conceive of the organization as a purely economic enterprise, a business with no moral obligations to patients.[29] The standards they discuss are not ethical principles, but management goals, such as economic efficiency, product quality, information dissemination and fair competition. A consensus on standards is unlikely unless these conflicting views are reconciled.

Problems with Business Ethics

Business ethics in the United States deal with the ethical conduct of business in a competitive marketplace.[30] The ethical principles governing business are designed to promote fair competition. These include honesty, truthfulness and keeping promises. More specific principles give content to these general principles. For example, businesspeople should avoid disseminating information that is false or misleading, and avoid exploiting relationships for personal gain.

Fair competition assumes some measure of equality among those who do business, and seeks to assure conditions in which people are free to make voluntary choices to buy or sell goods or services. Medical ethics, in contrast, assumes significant inequality in knowledge and skill between physicians and patients. For this reason, physicians have been found to have a type of fiduciary obligation to their patients. Business organizations do not have fiduciary obligations to their customers. Their fiduciary obligations are to their shareholders, in the case of investor-owned, for-profit enterprises,[31] or to the state, in the case of nonprofit organizations. Investor-owned businesses are expected to preserve their assets to accomplish the organization's business purpose and to provide a financial return to investors. Non-profit organizations must also use their resources to accomplish a stated noncommercial purpose.

MCOs face difficulties when achievement of their mission to provide medical care conflicts with their obligation to preserve their assets. This is especially true in the case of for-profit MCOs, which may be under pressure to maintain stock prices and to pay dividends. Some commercial organizations have attempted to adopt socially responsible corporate policies, such as producing or using products that do not harm the environment. Often, such products are both popular and profitable, so that the company can satisfy both its customers and its shareholders. Similarly, many MCOs hope that patient satisfaction will attract new subscribers and, hence, sufficient revenues to yield a satisfactory return to investors. Investors or shareholders of an MCO, however, are rarely the same people as those enrolled in the health plan. If an MCO's financial goals conflict with its service methods, little in the field of business ethics argues for giving subscribers priority.

Stanley Reiser offers the following values to guide health care institutions: humaneness, reciprocal benefit, trust, fairness, dignity, gratitude, service and stewardship.[32] Apart from fairness, such values are not generally included in discussions of business ethics. Richard DeGeorge describes American business values as freedom (to buy and sell), profit, fairness (including honesty and truthfulness), equal opportunity, and pragmatism or efficiency.[33] Some of Reiser's values may be incompatible with achieving the MCO's financial goals. For example, his concept of reciprocal benefit restrains institutions from actions that harm some to benefit others. MCOs, however, may have to allocate their resources in ways that explicitly harm some patients or providers to benefit others, so as to use resources efficiently to provide the most services to an entire enrollee population. The notion of service, or the obligation to use one's talents to benefit others rather than to expect rewards for labor, is similarly problematic. MCOs typically assume the opposite; they frequently use financial rewards and penalties to influence physician behavior, for example. In addition, humaneness, which encompasses compassion for people, may work against cost control, especially where compassion favors providing treatment that is not covered by a health plan. Although these values seem relevant to providing medical care (and appear to be derived from principles used in medical ethics), more sophisticated concepts are necessary if they are to be incorporated into standards that provide concrete guidance to MCOs.

Few business ethics texts even discuss organizations that deliver medical care. Most tend to focus on ethical principles for individual personal conduct, rather than the actions or policies of an organization.[34] The American College of Healthcare Executives (ACHE) has perhaps the best code of ethics for the behavior of health care executives.[35] Its preamble states that because "every management decision affects the health and well-being of both individuals and communities," health care executives "must safeguard and foster the rights, interests, and prerogatives of patients, clients or others served." Yet the code's normative responsibilities are primarily duties of honesty, such as conducting all professional activities with "honesty, integrity, respect, fairness, and good faith," being truthful and avoiding "information that is false, misleading, and deceptive or information that would create unreasonable expectation," avoiding "the exploitation of professional relationships for personal gain," and creating "institutional safeguards to prevent discriminatory organizational practices."

The ACHE Code makes clear that executives have a responsibility to the organization as well as to patients, noting that they should respect the customs of patients "consistent with the organization's philosophy." Obligations to provide health care services may be limited by available resources. Although executives are to assure "a resource allocation process that considers ethical ramifications," the code does not indicate what ethical principles might be relevant.[36] The fundamental question for managers is whether their responsibilities to the organization supersede any responsibilities to the patients served by the organization. In other words, when the organization's financial needs conflict with the needs of patients, does the manager have an ethical obligation to give patient needs priority? Unfortunately, existing codes of ethics do not answer this question. Most imply that constraints on organizational resources also constrain obligations to patients.[37]

It is possible that ethical management principles would bar organizations from excluding physicians who generate high costs by providing appropriate care to their patients. After all, if the organization's mission is to provide appropriate care to its patient population, its employed or contracting physicians cannot be faulted for achieving that mission. This would support recommendations that MCOs evaluate physician performance solely on the basis of quality of care, without regard to the quantity or cost of services generated.[38] At the same time, the organization needs to preserve itself; and if the cost of providing appropriate care became unreasonable, even a principle requiring fair treatment of physicians might not override the financial imperative of self-preservation. In the absence of any standard for determining the proportion of resources that should be devoted to patient care and for what an appropriate level of care should be, existing principles are not likely to resolve such conflicts. Moreover, fair treatment of physicians and employees would not require retaining subscribers whose illnesses were costly to treat. Thus, even ethical management principles are unlikely to prevent organizations from limiting medical benefits or excluding patients in the absence of other principles defining an obligation to provide care.

Even if codes of ethics for managers contained more specific normative principles, it is not clear how effective they would be in the face of countervailing financial pressure. No formal rules regulate the conduct of business managers. The ACHE's only sanction for violations of its code is expulsion from the ACHE, which does not necessarily affect an offender's ability to work. In contrast, a violation of the American Medical Association's *Principles of Medical Ethics,*[39] could result in a complaint to the board of registration, which has the power to revoke a physician's license to practice medicine, even if such sanctions are rarely invoked in practice.

Ethical Obligations to Patients/Enrollees

Although patients may view their health plan as an assurance of medical care, their legal relationship to an MCO is based on contract principles developed for application in the marketplace of consumer goods. The conditions for an enforceable contract are: an exchange of promises, a fair bargaining process (no coercion), and a meeting of the minds.[40] A relationship based on contract principles is fundamentally different from one based on trust or fiduciary obligations. For example, a physician has an ethical obligation to act in the patient's best interest, while a party to a contract need only perform according to the contract. Thus, in a contractual relationship, an MCO that does not provide care that is not promised in the contract does not treat patients unjustly, even if the care is necessary and appropriate.

While physicians have a duty to treat all patients equally, no contract principle requires that all contracts be the same. Thus, two patients with the same illness who are covered by different health plans may receive quite different treatment. In business ethics, the principle of honesty undoubtedly requires MCOs to inform prospective subscribers of the contract terms, but no principle insists that the contract contain specific benefits or be consistent with other contracts. Contract variations may violate some conceptions of justice, yet they are entirely consistent with market values and the goals of competition among health plans.

Fair competition is premised on the freedom of consumers to choose what goods and services to buy. In today's medical marketplace, consumer choice is advocated not only as a valuable freedom in itself, but also as a means to force MCOs to offer quality medical care. It is notable, therefore, that patient choice has all but disappeared from the goals of managed care.[41] If care is managed, then, by definition, the patient is not free to choose what care he or she gets. The American Heritage Dictionary, for example, defines *manage* as "to direct or control the use of; to exert control over; make submissive to one's authority, discipline, or persuasion."[42] The purpose of managing care is to eliminate choices that are wasteful, harmful or too expensive. Patient choice is not always desirable from society's perspective, because patients sometimes make unwise choices and want unnecessary or even harmful treatment. Managed care's cost-control mechanisms are designed to eliminate certain choices or to influence patients (by means of deductibles and copayments, for example) to choose specific (usually less expensive) types of care.[43] In the ideal world, good management will result in better care for patients, but it will not encourage patient choice.

Of course, managed care was never intended to promote patient choice of care. Rather, "choice" here is the choice of which health care plan to buy or "join."[44] If patients are consumers or customers, then the product is the health plan – that package of insured services paid for by the insurer, subject to deductibles, copayments, caps, and other limits. The organization's primary relationship to its patients is that of an insurer to an insured, not of a health care provider to a patient.[45] This is underscored by the insurance terminology for patients: subscribers, enrollees or, most recently, covered lives.

Advocates of competition among health plans have argued that rational people will choose the health plan that suits their needs.[46] They assume that, when people choose a plan, they have deliberately and necessarily chosen its doctors, nurses, practice patterns, administrative procedures, and benefits package – everything about their health care. A choice to buy a cheaper plan entails assuming the risk that some services will not be covered. For this reason, they conclude, patients must live (or die) with their choices – that is, what the health plan contract provides. This conclusion is based on false assumptions. The most obvious is that people make rational choices about their health care. Even if people could make rational choices about their health care, there are at least three practical problems with assuming that choosing a health plan satisfies the requirements of choice.

First, most patients do not choose their health plans; their employers do. The vast majority of Americans with health insurance get it through their employers.[47] The insurer's primary customers are employers, not individual patients. A recent survey found that among companies with fewer than 50 employees and with employee health insurance, 86% offered only one plan.[48] Sixty percent of larger firms offered no choice. The number of employers who offer plans that are closed panel HMOs or limited panel preferred provider organizations (PPOs) is increasing.[49] MCO growth rates are expected to continue over the next few years as government programs like Medicare and Medicaid encourage more beneficiaries to join managed care plans.[50] Thus, the number of patients who have not merely a limited choice of plans, but no choice of plans, is increasing.

A recent Commonwealth Fund study of 3,000 employees in Boston, Los Angeles and Miami found that 29% of respondents in managed care plans did not have the choice of enrolling in a FFS plan.[51] Those without such a choice reported more dissatisfaction with their plans than those who did.[52] Almost half of the employees had changed plans in the past three years, and of those, nearly three-fourths did so involuntarily. Employees who changed health plans were often forced to change physicians as well: 48% of HMO enrollees and 29% of PPO enrollees, compared to 12% of FFS patients.

If patients are not choosing the plans they join, it cannot be said that they are freely entering into a contract by which they should be bound. Of course, they could "choose" not to join the employer's plan, but for many employees, such a "choice" is unaffordable. Furthermore, people whose employers do not offer health insurance may have little or no choice of plans they can afford.

A second reason why patients do not choose their health plans in practice is that patients rarely know exactly what benefits their plans offer when they must choose them. It is the rare patient who fully understands a benefit contract or appreciates what it means to "choose" a health plan. Contracts are frequently revised and may not even be available to subscribers in final form until several months into the contract year. Information about plans is ordinarily summarized in general terms in brochures distributed to employees or prospective subscribers.[53] Summaries are clearest on how to choose a physician, where services are and are not available, and the amounts of copayments and deductibles. Benefits are usually described generically as hospital care, physicians' services and laboratory services, for example. Typically, mention is made of the fact that the plan covers "medically necessary" services, but subscribers may not appreciate that the term *medically necessary* serves as a limitation on coverage. It is often difficult to know what particular kinds of treatment are covered until a patient gets sick and needs specific services.[54] Then, it is too late: patients are not likely to be able to change plans at that time, either because they do not get sick during the annual plan enrollment period or because any new plan they join may exclude coverage for their now-preexisting illness, at least for the period in which they need treatment. Thus, much of the information necessary for a rational choice is not available when the choice must be made.

Finally, many patients do not want to be bound by their contracts. Even if patients had perfect information and actually chose their health plans, they would not necessarily want contract exclusions enforced when they get sick. "A deal is a deal" is not a palatable response to a dying patient who cannot afford the recommended treatment. People who appear to be rational consumers when they enroll in a health plan may change their minds when they need treatment. Many are surprised to find that, contrary to their expectations, their health plan does not cover the care they need or desire.[55] Even those who might have appreciated that the plan would not cover certain kinds of care (or did not want to pay for it), such as experimental treatment, may consider the contract unfair if the experiment offers their only chance for survival.

Patients may be especially likely to consider benefit denials unfair in a competitive environment where a wide variety of health plans offer different benefits; patients know that other health plans provide the desired care to their subscribers. Even where benefits are the same, different insurers may interpret them differently, resulting in inconsistent benefit determinations.[56] Many patients are likely to perceive such variation not as healthy variety in a free marketplace, but as arbitrary and unfair rationing by their health plan.[57] Given recent publicity about high profits earned by many HMOs and about multimillion-dollar compensation paid to their chief executive officers, subscribers may also believe that different treatment is based on corporate greed, not on individual patient needs.[58] This is not to suggest that patients are entitled to whatever care they want, but rather that they may want it, regardless of what their health plan covers or of the likely effectiveness of the desired treatment.[59]

The circumstances in which individuals enroll in health plans today are significantly removed from the basic conditions for fair and enforceable contracts contemplated by law. Yet, in spite of deviations from the ideal, courts have not questioned the validity of such contracts. Neither have they hesitated to enforce contract exclusions (denying medical benefits to patients) when their terms were clear.[60] Although enforcement has been inconsistent, courts have most commonly refused to enforce coverage exclusions on the grounds that the contract language was ambiguous or the treatment at issue was not necessarily excluded by explicit language. Thus, it seems unlikely that patients could successfully claim that their health plans are invalid.

Of course, ethical standards may demand more than law requires. Thus, whether making patients abide by the terms of their health plans is fair or unfair depends on how fairly the plans themselves are structured. But what should count as a fair structure? What choices ought to be available to patients? Fundamentally, the search for standards of fairness is a quest for ethical principles that prescribe what kind of care patients should get. Medical ethics suggests that every patient is entitled to the best available care, but does not obligate anyone to provide that care if it is not paid for. Business ethics also does not obligate anyone to provide any particular care to anyone else, absent a contractual promise. An adequate answer requires more specific standards than either business or medical ethics offers.

GOALS FOR DEVELOPING STANDARDS

What might new ethical standards for MCOs look like? Several basic features appear necessary, but will require substantially more discussion, definition and clarification than can be offered here.

First, ethical standards for MCOs should recognize the organizations' medical responsibilities as well as their business functions. The organization has responsibility – as an organization – for providing health care to individual enrollees, and this responsibility should not be delegable to individuals, even though officers and staff should remain bound by their personal ethical obligations. MCOs should be held directly accountable to enrollees for the scope and quality of patient care, because patients are not customers in the usual sense. Because the MCO's mission is to finance and provide quality medical care, its business structures, policies and practices should facilitate and not hinder good care. Indeed, ethical standards should give priority to MCOs' medical mission.

Second, organizational standards should reflect ethical principles that apply to all human endeavors, such as fairness, honesty, truthfulness, respect for persons and justice. The principle of justice, which governs resource allocation, is especially relevant to MCOs because the very nature of managed care requires allocating resources for the benefit of all members of a group. MCOs must marshal sufficient resources (both human and financial) to care for an entire patient population. In this respect, MCOs differ from other commercial enterprises that do not attempt to allocate their products or services among their potential customers. While physicians may act as patient advocates, the organization's purpose is to ensure that *all* of its enrollees receive appropriate care. Obvious potential conflicts arise between being fair to a population and being fair to an individual patient. But reaching acceptable solutions is more likely when decisions are based on ethical principles of justice and respect for persons than when they are perceived to be based on financial self-interest.

Of course, reasonable people disagree on what justice requires and on what counts as a just allocation of resources.[61] A standard that allocates benefits according to patient need is as plausible as one that eliminates expensive, experimental therapies in order to provide more preventive services. Some proponents of market competition in health care also adopt a libertarian view of justice that does not require any particular distribution of services. In this view, the principles of fair contracting are sufficient to create just allocation of resources, without regard to who receives what services or why. This latter approach, in effect, argues against any ethical standard that seeks to achieve a more equal distribution of services or benefits.

An even greater difficulty with just allocation as an ethical standard for MCOs is that it applies only to the organization itself. Although one MCO may produce a just distribution of resources across its own subscribers, it does not affect those in other plans or those without health insurance, so that the allocation of resources throughout society may remain quite unjust. One organization cannot be expected to solve the inequities of society as a whole, but society should recognize that organizations whose standards are entirely inward-looking are not likely to produce a fairer health care system.

The principles of honesty and fairness suggest that MCOs should fully and completely disclose the terms and conditions of the contracts they offer, especially in a market system that depends on consumer demand. At a minimum, this requires telling current and potential enrollees (and the public) what the plan does and does not provide, the specific conditions in which services will be made available, and ensuring that patients are not coerced into a particular plan.[62] An obligation on the MCO's part for even more extensive disclosure is supported by traditional business ethics and assumptions about market transactions. Fair competition requires informed consumers. Disclosure is a competitive market method of promoting informed consumer choice.

Full disclosure is also supported, analogously, by the doctrine of informed consent.[63] If a subscriber is validly to consent to join a health plan (and to be bound by its terms), then the MCO – the entity with the relevant information – should have a duty to disclose all information relevant to the subscriber's decision. This should include detailed information on the specific treatments that are and are not covered for particular medical conditions, the criteria for making decisions about new or innovative therapies, the MCO's history of approving or denying claims for treatment, and procedures for challenging treatment denials. In addition, the MCO should disclose all financial arrangements with providers, including affiliated physicians and hospitals, and the organization's officers and employees.[64] Standard formats for presenting information should be developed to enable consumers to compare different health plans. The MCO should also ensure that its officers, employees and health care practitioners are equally open and honest with patients. Full disclosure is intended to move the relationship between MCOs and patients closer to one of fair bargaining, so that patients can actually begin to choose.[65]

There are limits to the utility of information disclosure, however.[66] Not everyone will see or understand the information provided. More importantly, many consumers do not have the freedom to act on the information or to bargain at all. Their employer may offer only one plan, and they may not be able to afford the plan they prefer. The current market does not include any mechanism for such consumers to pressure MCOs to change their policies.[67] Thus, full disclosure is necessary, but insufficient to foster a fair contractual relationship.

MCOs that distinguish themselves by adhering to ethical standards may find that they are penalized in the marketplace. For most commercial enterprises, customer satisfaction produces increased revenues and profits and higher stock values. Patient satisfaction, however, may be associated with more services that cost a for-profit MCO revenues and reduce stock prices. A competitive market is likely to discourage MCOs from seeking subscribers who are likely to need expensive medical care (or from contracting with their physicians). This means that a competitive market will not provide universal health insurance coverage. Some regulation may be necessary to permit MCOs to compete without abandoning their ethical standards. For example, were all companies required to enroll individuals regardless of their medical conditions (assuming a fair distribution of either high-risk patients or premium adjustments, with or without financial assistance from government), MCOs would be free to compete on quality of care, including patient satisfaction. Universal coverage would undoubtedly reduce the feasible profit margin for all companies, but the pressure to sacrifice patient welfare for cost control would be substantially diminished. In such circumstances, ethical standards promoting patient welfare could enhance a company's competitive position. Thus, a regulated market that removes or reduces incentives to compete for profits is more likely to encourage the adoption of ethical standards that protect patients.

CONCLUSION

MCOs combine insurance, management and health care delivery. They face conflicts between their financial incentives and their mission (or potential ethical duty) to provide appropriate care that are analogous to the conflicts faced by physicians in MCOs. The difference between the organizations and the physicians (and other professionals) is that neither the manager nor the organization has any significant history of ethical obligations that counter inappropriate financial incentives. Patients and physicians may wish to judge MCOs by ethical standards that were created for individual physicians and nurses, but the market in which MCOs operate does not use those standards. Those who argue that MCOs should operate like efficient businesses in the competitive marketplace are, in effect, arguing for no standards at all. A free-market approach stresses organizing and delivering health care in an economically efficient, value-free way. This effectively precludes the imposition of normative values on MCOs.

In absence of standards that address MCOs' business and medical functions, we may be left with two incompatible sets of standards – one for business and one for medicine. Scholars have begun to rethink conceptions of medical ethics for physicians in MCOs. It is time to rethink business ethics for MCOs. If business ethics do not recognize an organizational commitment to patient welfare, conflicts between physicians and managers, and managers and patients may be exacerbated, pitting financial power against patient welfare. In such circumstances, it is not cynical to fear that financial pressure may overwhelm patient welfare, leaving companies who risk too much money to provide services to patients at a competitive disadvantage or out of business.

MCOs should not have to choose between ethics and money, but they do need a different set of standards from those of ordinary commercial enterprises. The challenge is to formulate new standards that apply to organizations, not just individuals, and that recognize and reconcile their business and medical functions. If such standards are to be more than idealistic goals, however, it may be necessary to regulate the market to make it possible for organizations to put such standards into practice.

KEY IDEAS IN THIS ARTICLE:

- The traditional principles that have applied to health practitioners in the delivery of medical care do not easily apply to managed care organizations (MCOs).

- While MCOs do provide medical care, they are also a business. In other words, MCOs, unlike other organizations, have both medical and business functions.

- There is little doubt that ethical principles are needed to guide the activities of MCOs. The difficulty is in specifying what those principles or standards should be, such that they take into account the dual business and medical functions of MCOs. Most proposed standards address one or the other function, but not both.

- Neither business nor medical ethics offers sufficient standards to provide guidance in addressing the difficult ethical issues faced by MCOs. The challenge is to formulate new standards that apply both to organizations and to individuals, and that recognize and reconcile MCOs' business and medical functions.

- There are three goals for developing new standards. They should (1) recognize the dual functions of MCOs, perhaps giving priority to the medical function; (2) reflect ethical principles that apply to all human endeavors, such as fairness, honesty, truthfulness, respect for persons, and justice; and (3) facilitate full disclosure of the terms and conditions of contracts.

A SUGGESTED PROCESS FOR REFLECTING ON THIS ARTICLE:

(See pages 234-254 for other processes that might better fit your specific goals and objectives.)

Identify three aspects or components of managed care as it exists in your institution, and develop one or more ethical standards to guide the activities related to that component, bearing in mind both the business and health-care delivery aspects of managed care.

Component of Managed Care	Ethical Standard(s)
1.	
2.	
3.	

Circulate the standards amongst the group. Review, discuss and revise each as needed. Are there areas of managed care in your institution that are not covered by these ethical standards/guidelines and should be? Create standards to address these areas as necessary.

Other Components/Aspects of Managed Care	Ethical Standards
1.	
2.	
3.	

What are likely consequences of implementing these ethical standards in your organization for both the business and healthcare realms? Consider both positive and negative consequences, short-and long-term. Are there any trade-offs that will need to be made? Are these trade-offs justified?

Ethical Standards	+ Consequences for Health Care Delivery	- Consequences for Health Care Delivery	+ Consequences for Business	- Consequences for Business
1.				
2.				
3.				

What will need to occur for these ethical standards to be successfully implemented? What obstacles might be encountered? What new structures or processes need to be put in place? How will these standards be communicated to associates of your organization? How, if at all, will these standards be communicated in any way to patients?

What might be the next steps in developing and implementing ethical standards for managed care in your institution?

ENDNOTES

1. Erik Eckholm, "While Congress Remains Silent, Health Care Transforms Itself," *New York Times,* Dec. 18, 1994, at 34.

2. John K. Iglehart, "The American Health Care System – Managed Care," *N. Engl. J. Med.,* 327 (1992): 743-47.

3. Marc A. Rodwin, "Conflicts in Managed Care," *N. Engl. J. Med.,* 332 (1995): 604-07.

4. Marc A. Rodwin, *Medicine, Money & Morals: Physicians' Conflicts of Interest* (New York: Oxford University Press, 1993); and Peter Franks, Carolyn M. Clancy, and Paul A. Nutting, "Gatekeeping Revisited – Protecting Patients from Overtreatment," *N. Engl. J. Med.,* 327 (1992): 424-29.

5. Edmund D. Pellegrino, "Words *Can* Hurt You: Some Reflections on the Metaphors of Managed Care," *Journal of the American Board of Family Practice,* 7 (1994): 505-10.

6. Committee on Child Health Financing, American Academy of Pediatrics, "Guiding Principles for Managed Care Arrangements for the Health Care of Infants, Children, Adolescents, and Young Adults," *Pediatrics,* 95 (1995): 613-15; Council on Ethical and Judicial Affairs, American Medical Association, "Ethical Issues in Managed Care," *JAMA,* 271 (1994): 1668-70; Mark H. Waymack, "Health Care as a Business: The Ethic of Hippocrates versus the Ethic of Managed Care," *Business & Professional Ethics Journal,* 9, nos. 3-4 (1990): 69-78; and Susan M. Wolf, "Health Care Reform and the Future of Physician Ethics," *Hastings Center Report,* 24, no. 2 (1994): 28-41.

7. Carolyn M. Clancy and Howard Brody, "Managed Care – Jekyll or Hyde?," *JAMA,* 273 (1995): 338-39.

8. The percentage of MCOs that are for-profit companies grew from 18% in 1982 to 67% in 1988. See Karen Davis et al., *Health Care Cost Containment* (Baltimore: Johns Hopkins University Press, 1990).

9. The White House Domestic Policy Council, *The President's Health Security Plan. The Clinton Blueprint* (New York: Times Books, 1993): at 11-12.

10. As Sager has noted, managed care, in the form of employee group health organizations, was considered a radical (even socialist) innovation before and after World War II. See Alan Sager, "Reforming Managed Care: More Benefits – Fewer Costs," presented at the conference "Ethics of Managed Care: Values, Conflicts, and Resolutions," Boston University School of Public Health, Boston, Massachusetts, December 9, 1994. Group Health of Puget Sound, the Health Insurance Plan of New York, and the Kaiser-Permanente Medical Care Program have provided comprehensive care at a relatively reasonable cost to large groups of employees for at least 50 years. See John G. Smillie, *Can Physicians Manage the Quality and Costs of Medical Care? The Story of the Permanente Group* (New York: McGraw-Hill, 1991).

11. Theodore R. Marmor and Jonathan Oberiander, "A Citizen's Guide to the Healthcare Reform Debate," *Yale Journal on Regulation,* 11 (1994): 495-506.

12. Stephen M. Shortell, Robin R. Gillies, and David A. Anderson, "The New World of Managed Care: Creating Organized Delivery Systems," *Health Affairs,* 13, no. 4 (1994): 46-64 and Alain C. Enthoven, "The History and Principles of Managed Competition," *Health Affairs,* 12, supp. (1993): 24-48.

13. Paul Starr, "Look Who's Talking Health Care Reform Now," *New York Times Magazine,* Sept. 3, 1995, at 42-43.

14. R.H. Miller and Harold S. Luft, "Managed Care Plan Performance Since 1980: A Literature Analysis," *JAMA,* 271 (1995): 1512-19.

15. Congressional Budget Office, *The Effects of Managed Care and Managed Competition, CBO Memorandum* (Washington, D.C.: Congressional Budget Office, Feb. 1995);

Theodore R. Marmor and Jerry L. Mashaw, "Conceptualizing, Estimating, and Reforming Fraud, Waste, and Abuse in Healthcare Spending," *Yale Journal on Regulation*, 11 (1994): 455-94; William B. Schwartz and Daniel N. Mendelson, "Eliminating Waste and Inefficiency Can Do Little to Contain Costs," *Health Affairs*, 13, no. 1 (1994); 223-35; and Henry Aaron and William B. Schwarz, "Rationing Health Care: The Choice Before Us," *Science*, 247 (1990): 418-22.

16. See Iglehart, *supra* note 2.

17. Institute of Medicine, Bradford H. Gray and Marilyn J. Field, eds. *Controlling Costs and Changing Patient Care? The Role of Utilization Management* (Washington D.C.: National Academy Press, 1989); Alan L. Hillman, Mark V. Pauly, and Joseph J. Kerstein, "How Do Financial Incentives Affect Physicians' Clinical Decisions and the Financial Performance of Health Maintenance Organizations?," *N. Engl. J. Med.*, 321 (1989): 87-92; and Rodwin, *supra* note 4.

18. Donald W. Light, "The Practice and Ethics of Risk-Rated Health Insurance," *JAMA*, 267 (1992): 2503-08.

19. Several states have considered legislation prohibiting insurers from excluding coverage of preexisting medical conditions (completely or for a limited time period). In general, the insurance industry has opposed such legislation.

20. James Morone, "The Ironic Flaw in Health Care Competition: The Politics of Markets," in Richard J. Arnould et al., eds., *Competitive Approaches to Health Care Reform* (Washington, D.C.: Urban Institute Press, 1993): 207-22; Gerald W. Grumet, "Health Care Rationing Through Inconvenience: The Third Party's Secret Weapon," *N. Engl. J. Med.*, 321 (1989): 607-11; U.S. Inspector General, *Beneficiary Perspectives of Medicare Risk HMOs* (Washington, D.C.: Dept. of Health and Human Services, OEI-06-91-00730, 1995); and Robert Blendon, *Sick People in Managed Care Have Difficulty Getting Services and Treatment* (Princeton: Robert Wood Johnson Foundation, 1995).

21. Wendy K. Mariner, "Patients' Rights after Health Care Reform: Who Decides What is Medically Necessary?" *American Journal of Public Health*, 84 (1994): 1515-20.

22. U.S. Congress, Office of Technology Assessment, *Identifying Health Technologies That Work: Searching for Evidence* (Washington, D.C.: Government Printing Office, OTA-H-608, Sept. 1994); and Wendy K. Mariner, "Outcomes Assessment in Health Care Reform: Promise and Limitations," *American Journal of Law & Medicine*, XX (1994): 37-57.

23. Tom Beauchamp and LeRoy Walters, *Contemporary Issues in Bioethics* (Belmont: Wadsworth, 4th ed., 1994). The concept of medical ethics itself is subject to different interpretations. See Michael A. Grodin, "Introduction: The Historical and Philosophical Roots of Bioethics," in Michael A. Grodin, ed., *Meta Medical Ethics: The Philosophical Foundations of Bioethics* (Dordrecht: Kluwer, 1995): at 1-26.

24. See Wolf, *supra* note 6.

25. George J. Annas, "Transferring the Ethical Hot Potato," *Hastings Center Report*, 17, no. 1 (1987): 20-21. With respect to whether corporations in general are moral entities, compare Milton Friedman, "The Social Responsibility of Business Is to Increase its Profits," *New York Times Magazine*, Sept. 13, 1970, at 32-33, 122, 124, 126; Herbert A. Simon, *Administrative Behavior* (New York: Free Press, 1965) (arguing that corporations cannot be held morally responsible); and Jon Ladd, "Morality and the Ideal of Rationality in Formal Organizations," *The Monist*, 54 (1970): 488-516 (arguing for corporate responsibility). For general discussions of the debate, see Peter A. French, *Collective and Corporate Responsibility* (New York: Columbia Universiey Press, 1984); and Hugh Curtier, ed., *Shame, Responsibility and the Corporation* (New York: Haven, 1986).

26. Richard T. DeGeorge, *Business Ethics* (New York: Macmillan, 4th ed., 1995): at 127.

27. Legal obligations have been a significant source of ethical standards for business. See Paul Steidlmeier, *People and Profits: The Ethics of Capitalism* (Englewood Cliffs: Prentice Hall 1992). at 14; and John R. Boatright, *Ethics and the Conduct of Business* (Englewood Cliffs: Prentice Hall, 1993): at 386. Federal antitrust legislation, such as the Sherman Act and the Robinson-Patman Act, were arguably efforts to impose ethical standards of fair

competition on industry, and law is often seen as the "guardian of business ethics." See Verne E. Henderson, *What's Ethical in Business* (New York: McGraw-Hill, 1992): at 7.

28. Daniel P. Sulmasy, "Physicians, Cost Control and Ethics," *Annals of Internal Medicine,* 116 (1992): 920-26; Gail Povar and John Moreno, "Hippocrates and the Health Maintenance Organization," *Annals of Internal Medicine,* 109 (1988): 419-24; Council on Ethical and Judicial Affairs, *supra* note 6; Pellegrino, *supra* note 5; and Wolf, *supra* note 6.

29. Lester C. Thurow, "Medicine Versus Economics," *N. Engl. J. Med.,* 313 (1985): 611-14.

30. See, for example, DeGeorge, *supra* note 26; James P. Wilbur, *The Moral Foundations of Business Practice* (Lanham: University Press of America, 1992); Ronald M. Green, *The Ethical Manager: A New Method for Business Ethics* (New York: Macmillan, 1994); Ronald Berenbeim, *Corporate Ethics* (New York: Conference Board, 1992); Karen Paul, ed., *Business Environment and Business Ethics* (Cambridge: Ballinger, 1987) and Henderson, *supra* note 27.

31. See Boatright, *supra* note 27, at 386; and DeGeorge, *supra* note 26.

32. Stanley Joel Reiser, "The Ethical Life of Health Care Organizations," *Hastings Center Report,* 24, no. 6 (1994): 28-35.

33. See DeGeorge, *supra* note 26. Steidlmeier has summarized American business values as follows: "(1) protecting the interests of property owners by promoting efficiency, reducing costs, and thereby increasing profits; (2) encouraging respect for the rights of property owners; (3) refraining from anticompetitive activities; (4) guarding the freedom of labor, owners, and customers; (5) discouraging government interference; (6) developing personal honesty, responsibility and industriousness; and (7) encouraging private contributions to charity." See Steidlmeier, *supra* note 27.

34. See, for example, Kurt Darr, *Ethics in Health Services Management* (Baltimore: Health Professions Press, 2d ed., 1993), which is directed at developing a personal ethic for individual managers.

35. American College of Healthcare Executives, *Codes of Ethics* (1988).

36. The American College of Health Care Administrators' *Code of Ethics* requires the administrator to "strive to provide to all those entrusted to his or her care the highest quality or appropriate services possible *in light of resources or other constraints.*" See The American College of Health Care Administrators, *Code of Ethics* (1989) (emphasis added). Even the Joint Commission on Accreditation of Healthcare Organizations, which requires hospitals to have a mechanism for considering ethical issues in patient care, qualifies its requirement by providing that the hospital reasonably respond to a patient's need for treatment "within the hospital's capacity." See Joint Commission on Accreditation of Healthcare Organizations, 199: *Accreditation Manual for Hospitals, Vol. I Standards* (Oakbrook Terrace: JCAHO, 1994).

37. The Group Health Association of America has proposed some standards for managed care and health plans, but these deal with financial solvency requirements (common in insurance regulation), patient confidentiality, and some consumer protections. See John K. Iglehart, "The Struggle Between Managed Care and Fee-for-Service Practice," *N. Engl. J. Med.,* 331 (1994): 63-67.

38. See Council on Ethical and Judicial Affairs, *supra* note 6.

39. American Medical Association, *Principles of Medical Ethics* (Chicago: American Medical Association, 1980).

40. Joseph M. Perillo, *Corbin on Contracts* (St. Paul: West, vol. 1, 1993).

41. MCOs are increasingly offering preferred provider or point of service plans that permit enrollees to obtain service outside the plan's network of providers for a larger copayment or deductible. Such plans appear to be a response to enrollee demand for greater freedom to choose physicians and services.

42. *American Heritage Dictionary* (Boston: Houghton Mifflin, 1978): at 792.

43. Health plans that offer services through independent practice association (IPAs) preserve greater choice of physicians for enrollees than do staff model HMOs, for example.

Historically, however, IPAs have produced smaller cost savings for health plans. See Miller and Luft, *supra* note 14.

44. Alain C. Enthoven and Richard Kronick, "A Consumer-Choice Health Plan for the 1990's: Universal Health Insurance in a System Designed to Promote Quality and Economy," *N. Engl. J. Med.,* 320 (1989): 29-37.

45. Of course, most MCOs also provide health care through providers in a widening array of organizational structures, including staff model HMOs, group practice HMOs, networks of IPAs, or other integrated services and preferred provider organizations.

46. Paul Starr, "The Framework of Health Care Reform," *N. Engl. J. Med.,* 329 (1993): 1666-72; Enthoven and Kronick, *supra* note 44; Mark A. Hall and Gerard F. Anderson, "Health Insurers' Assessment of Medical Necessity," *University of Pennsylvania Law Review,* 140 (1992): 1637-712; Paul T. Menzel, *Strong Medicine: The Ethical Rationing of Health Care* (New York; Oxford University Press, 1990); and David Eddy, "Clinical Decision Making: From Theory to Practice – Connecting Value and Costs – Whom Do We Ask and What Do We Ask Them?," *JAMA,* 264 (1990): 1737-39.

47. Employee Benefit Research Institute, *Sources of Health Insurance and Characteristics of the Uninsured: Analysis of the March 1993 Current Population Survey* (Washington, D.C.: EBRI, Jan. 1994).

48. Joel C. Cantor, Stephen H. Long, and M. Susan Marquis, "Private Employer-Based Health Insurance in Ten States," *Health Affairs,* 14, no. 2 (1995): 199-211. Smaller employers were more likely than larger to offer a FFS plan, but such plans were more likely to cover fewer benefits and to exclude preexisting conditions. Only about half of the smaller employers offered any health insurance at all.

49. Deborah Chollet, "Employer-Based Health Insurance in a Changing Work Force," *Health Affairs,* 13, no. 1 (1994): 327-36.

50. Christopher Georges, "Medicare Drive Toward Managed-Care System Could Turn Out to Produce a Costly Success," *Wall Street Journal,* July 31, 1995, at 16; and John K. Iglehart, "Medicaid and Managed Care," *N. Engl. J. Med.,* 322 (1995): 1727-31. Some states, like Tennessee, Florida and New York, have reported problems in moving Medicaid beneficiaries quickly into some managed care plans. See Ian Fisher, "Forced Marriage of Medicaid and Managed Care Hits Snags," *New York Times,* Aug. 28, 1995, at Bl, B5; and Martin Gottlieb, "The Managed Care Cure-All Shows its Flaws and Potential," *New York Times,* Oct. 1, 1995, at 1, 16.

51. Karen Davis et al., "Choice Matters: Enrollees' Views of Their Health Plans," *Health Affairs,* 14, no. 2 (1995): 99-112.

52. The Commonwealth Fund Survey found that among respondents who reported a serious illness, 45% of those in FFS medicine rated their plans as excellent, compared to 33% of those in managed care. *Id.*

53. The Employee Retirement Income Security Act, 29 U.S.C.S. §§55 1021-25 (1995), which governs employee group health insurance plans offered by employers, requires only that employees receive a summary of the plan, not the contract itself.

54. Describing covered benefits in detail would require extensive lists because appropriate treatment often depends significantly on individual medical conditions. See Ira Mark Ellman and Mark A. Hall, "Redefining the Terms of Insurance to Accommodate Varying Consumer Risk Preferences," *American Journal of Law & Medicine,* XX (1994): 187-201.

55. Recent examples of patients who claimed their health plan should have covered various treatments are described in a series of articles by Michael A. Hiltzik, David R. Olmos, and Barbara Marsh in *The Los Angeles Times,* Aug. 27-31, 1995.

56. U.S. General Accounting Office, *Medicare Part B: Inconsistent Denial Rates for Medical Necessity Across Six Carriers* (Washington, D.C.: GAO, GAO/T-PEMD-94-17, 1994); and General Accounting Office, *Medicare Part B: Regional Variation in Denial Rates for Medical Necessity* (Washington, D.C.: GAO, GAO/PEMD-95-10, 1994).

57. Wendy K. Mariner, "Rationing Health Care and the Need for Credible Scarcity: Why Americans Can't Say No," *American Journal of Public Health,* 85 (1995): 1439-45.

58. George Anders, "HMOs Paid Up Billions in Cash, Try to Decide What to Do With It," *Wall Street Journal,* Dec. 21, 1994, at Al, A5; and Milt Freudenheim, "Penny-pinching H.M.O.'s Showed Their Generosity in Executive Paychecks," *New York Times,* Apr. 11, 1995, at Dl, D4. In remarks to Congress on August 30, 1995, H. Ross Perot was reported to say, "If someone were to ask me what is my principal concern about H.M.O.'s, it's the giant concentration of power; it's the giant salaries. . . . You know, that doesn't look good to me." See Robert Pear, "Perot Tells Senate Committee It's Time to Get Experts' Opinion on Reining in Medicare," *New York Times,* Aug. 31, 1995, at B13.

59. See Mariner, *supra* note 57.

60. See, for example, *Fuja v. Benefit Trust Life Ins.* Co., 18 F3d 1405 (7th Cir. 1994).

61. For summaries of different conceptions of justice with respect to allocating health care resources, see John F. Kilner, "Allocation of Health-Care Resources," in Warren Thomas Reich, ed., *Encyclopedia of Bioethics* (New York: Simon & Schuster, vol. 4, 1995): at 1067-84; and President's Commission for the Study of Ethical Problems in Medicine and Biomedical and Behavioral Research, *Securing Access to Health Care: Report on the Ethical Implications of Differences in the Availability of Health Services* (Washington, D.C.: President's Commission, 1983).

62. Anderson et. al. have recommended objective assessments of technologies and therapies and better education to ensure that patients know what they are buying. Gerald F. Anderson, Mark A. Hall, and Earl P. Steinberg, "Medical Technology Assessment and Practice Guidelines: Their Day in Court," *American Journal of Public Health,* 83 (1993): 1635-39,

63. Ruth R. Faden and Tom L. Beauchamp, *A History and Theory of Informed Consent* (NewYork: Oxford University Press, 1986).

64. Ironically, capitation of physicians – the financial arrangement that has prompted the most concern about ethical standards – may be the least problematic method of payment. This is because capitation permits the MCO to avoid micromanaging patient care decisions in order to control costs. When the risk of financial loss is shifted to the physician, an MCO's financial self-interest rarely conflicts with patient welfare. It is the physician who faces a potential conflict. Physicians have a longer history of personal obligations to patients defined by medical ethics. Nonetheless, because the MCO is responsible for patient care, it should have a responsibility to calculate capitation payments that adequately provide for its patients. In addition, the MCO may be obligated to create different physician payment arrangements that reduce the potential conflict of interest.

65. Several states have introduced legislation to require the disclosure of certain information by MCOs, but the industry has generally opposed such regulation. Michael A. Hiltzik and David R. Olmos, "State Widely Criticized for Regulation of HMOs," *Los Angeles Times,* Aug. 28, 1995, at Al.

66. See Rodwin, *supra* note 4, at 212-22.

67. Yarmolinsky has noted, "Patients may be the only consumers who have to seek permission from someone else in order to obtain services." See Adam Yarmolinsky, "Supporting the Patient," *N. Engl. J. Med.,* 332 (1995): 602-03. In some instances, employees may be able to persuade their employers to offer a different health plan or to have the employer negotiate with an MCO to change the terms of the plan.

CHAPTER 10

ETHICALLY IMPORTANT DISTINCTIONS AMONG MANAGED CARE ORGANIZATIONS

Kate T. Christensen

DUE TO SOCIETY'S NEED TO CONTROL HEALTH CARE COSTS AND TO THE FAILURE of legislated health care reform, managed care is expanding at a rapid rate and will soon be the predominate form of health care delivery.[1] Plans by Congress to bring Medicare and Medicaid under managed care will further consolidate this trend.[2] Barring some legislative fiat, managed care is here to stay.

The term *managed care* describes a diverse set of organizational forms. Wide variations in approach, financing, physician involvement and philosophy exist among the different types of managed care organizations (MCOs). While many articles on the ethics of managed care acknowledge this variety, most analyses focus on the for-profit entities, paying less attention to the ethical distinctions among the different forms of managed care.[3] This paper discusses the key distinctions among MCO types, in particular the difference between for-profit and non-profit plans; the relationship of the physician to the MCO; the incentives used to control costs; the incentives that improve patient care; and the organizational features that nurture the principled practice of medicine.

KEY DISTINCTIONS AMONG MCOs

For-profit versus non-profit managed care

Although MCOs come in a bewildering array of structures, three crucial distinctions can be made among them: profit status, the relationship of physicians to the organization, and the nature of the capitation arrangement. The most important difference is between for-profit and non-profit health plans. For-profit plans make up the fastest growing segment of the managed care market, are growing at a much faster rate than the non-profits, and receive most of the business news attention.[4] Although all MCOs must generate surplus revenue to continue to operate, for-profit plans differ from non-profit in that they trade their shares publicly and are not governed by the rules of charitable organizations.[5] As a result, their administrative costs as a percentage of total income tends to be much higher. For-profit administrative costs often include extraordinarily large CEO salaries and bonuses, dividends to shareholders, and cash reserves for acquisition of competitors.[6] A recent survey in California revealed a wide range between the total administrative expenses of for-profit organizations, which run as high as 30.9% of total revenue, and non-profit organizations, like Kaiser Foundation Health Plan, Inc. in California, which run at 3.1%.[7] Other non-profit health plans also tend to have a larger share of income devoted to health services and a smaller profit/income ratio.[8] This difference becomes ethically relevant when we consider the pressure on physicians to limit health care costs. Subscriber premiums or dues are set by the marketplace and, because of direct competition between plans, the costs of the different plans tend to be very close. Therefore, in order to create more profit, the surplus is generated elsewhere. Part of it comes from reducing the amount spent on doctors, tests, treatments and hospitalization.[9] It stands to reason, then, that physicians in an MCO that has both less to spend on patient care and stockholders to please will be under more pressure to cut corners.[10] Corner-cutting, or erring on the side of doing less instead of more, is a reality now. Only future research will tell us whether such practices are having a negative impact on patient care.

PHYSICIANS AND THE MCO

The second relevant distinction between MCO types is the relationship of the physician to the organization,[11] which manifests itself in the various incentives to control patient care costs.[12] For physicians, incentives can influence their professional autonomy as well as their practice stability and quality of professional work life, which in turn impact the quality of patient care in a variety of ways.[13]

All health care delivery systems have financial incentives that can influence physician behavior. Under the traditional fee-for-service (FFS) model, physicians are rewarded financially for overtreating patients.[14] And because many patients believe that more health care is better health care, physicians have a further incentive to keep patients happy by doing more. This system (along with technological advances and increased public expectations) has led to spiraling health care costs and, at times, iatrogenic harm to patients. Few tests or procedures are entirely risk-free, and incidental findings can cause unnecessary anxiety as well as further tests or procedures. Although FFS allows physicians more practice and administrative

Table 1. The Financial Relationship of the Physician to the MCO.			
Practice Type	**Relationship of Physician to MCO**	**Physician Payment**	**Physician Involvement in QA/UR**
PPO	Physicians contract with HMO	Discounted FFS	High
IPA/Network	Physicians contract with MCOs through IPA	Usually capitation	High
Group Model	Group contacts with MCO	Capitation to group; salary with various incentives	High
Staff Model	Physician is employee of MCO	Salary with various incentives	Low

Table 2. Spectrum of Physician Incentives*		
	Traditional FFS	**Managed Care**
Compensation:	Fee per service rendered	Fee per person enrolled (capitation)
General Incentive:	Do more, get more	Do less, get more
Examples of Specific Financial Incentives	Direct reimbursement for patient care; income from laboratory or radiology services; partnership in hospital	Withhold part of income; capitation, direct or diffused; bonuses; threat of deselection
*This chart is abstract, in that it does not take into account the many variations on these basic themes among MCOs.		

autonomy than any other system, this system is rapidly withering in the face of the massive growth and consolidation of MCOs, as well as the cost-containment measures to limit Medicare, and Medicaid reimbursements. Many FFS physicians are now contracting with a variety of MCOs.[15]

For many years, Kaiser Permanente was the only large-scale alternative to FFS in the United States. Now MCOs include a growing array of reimbursement and health care delivery systems. Many MCOs offer a number of different products to enrollees and employers, giving each a choice from a menu of managed care and traditional indemnity plans. The basic forms currently are the independent practice associations (IPAs), preferred provider organizations (PPOs), the group model HMOs (like Kaiser Permanente), and the staff model HMOs.

PPO physicians contract with the MCO, and are paid on an FFS basis (see Table 1). Fees are usually discounted deeply by the health plan and, as a result, many FFS physicians have experienced declining incomes in the last five years.[16] Physicians in PPOs typically have contracts with a number of different MCOs and some indemnity plans. Because these physicians are still paid per service rendered, an inherent incentive arises to generate more health care costs by seeing patients more often and/or by ordering more tests and interventions (see Table 2).[17] These physicians also are exposed to sudden changes in their relationship with the health plan, such as contract termination and the subsequent loss of covered patients. Therefore, income security is lowest for this group of physicians, in particular for the subspecialists. Physicians in IPAs also contract with one or more MCOs, but are given organizational coherence and negotiating power by the practice association. They are usually reimbursed on a capitated basis.[18]

In the group model HMO, the physician is part of a group that contracts with the HMO. Instead of receiving a fee for each service rendered, the group is paid a capitated amount by the health plan in advance of providing patient care services. The physicians are typically paid a basic salary plus a variety of financial incentives, such as bonuses. In contrast, physicians in staff model HMOs are employees of the MCO. They are salaried, and are also paid a variety of incentives – similar to group model physicians – designed to promote cost-effective medical care. Job security is often low in this group, because of the employee status of the physicians. Some predict that the majority of physicians will be working for staff model HMOs in the future.[19]

Financial incentives common to many MCOs are the payment of bonuses from any unspent funds and withholding of portions of income, which may be paid out at the end of the year if certain cost-containment targets are met. Such targets may include keeping hospital utilization below a certain rate or limiting referrals to specialists. The larger the amount of the withheld income, the stronger the incentive to toe the line.[20] Laboratory and radiology costs are frequently deducted from the pooled funds as well.[21] In all but the group model HMOs, the threat of job loss or loss of one's patients also serves as a potent incentive to adhere to the MCO's rules.

Another significant aspect of the relationship of physicians to MCOs is the degree of control physicians have over the administrative and clinical aspects of their practices. In IPAs and PPOs income security may be low, but physician autonomy over medical practice is high, because physicians retain much of the traditional FFS prerogatives and practice format. Although practice autonomy is more restricted in group model HMOs than in IPAs or PPOs, physicians in IPAs, PPOs and group model HMOs typically manage their own utilization review, quality assurance and cost controls. Practice autonomy is usually lowest in the staff model HMOs, where utilization review and cost controls are usually managed and implemented by health plan administrators. Experience to date indicates that when control over the clinical aspects of practice rests with nonphysician administrators, the quality of patient care is threatened and physician morale plummets.[22]

Many physicians are happy to relinquish administrative responsibility for their medical practices, but are uncomfortable with losing control over the clinical aspects, such as utilization and quality management. Physicians in MCOs know that utilization review can be benign or malignant, depending on who is doing it and to what end. This is the nightmare of utilization review: a stranger in another city, who has no clinical experience, calls the doctor and tells her to discharge a patient, or denies approval for a test the physician deems necessary. When used in this way, utilization review can function as a barrier to patient care.[23] Physicians' job stress can be significantly increased by having to negotiate these hurdles on behalf of their patients.[24] That situation also raises a direct conflict of interest between physicians' duty to provide good patient care and their own financial health.[25]

However, when managed and implemented by physicians, utilization review can both promote better patient care (by minimizing unnecessary treatments or hospital stays) and save money. Utilization review should not put up barriers to good patient care and, in the hands of physicians, it is less likely to do so.[26]

Similarly, practice guidelines can be imposed on physicians, as in many staff model MCOs, or developed and implemented by physicians, as in the group model MCOs.[27] When used inappropriately, such guidelines are applied as standards to measure, reward and punish physician behavior.[28] But with physician involvement, this process serves as a useful extension of peer review, and helps to maintain a high quality of care. When physicians are involved in the development and implementation of practice guidelines, it is less likely that they will mistake guidelines for standards (which require more stringent outcomes studies and stricter enforcement)[29] and inappropriately use the guidelines to reward and punish.

CAPITATION

Another useful distinction among MCOs is the way members' premiums are distributed to the physicians.[30] Capitation forms the core financial process in all of the systems discussed above. In a capitated system, the pool of funds for the provision of services is collected by the health plan and then distributed in various ways, often called *risk sharing*. Some plans give a physician group the money (less administrative costs and, if applicable, profit), and the money is kept in a central pool to pay for health care services. Other plans give the funds to the physicians, or to small physician groups, and the physicians then keep whatever is left at the end of the period (monthly, quarterly or yearly). The more individualized the capitation arrangement is in relation to the physician, the greater the ethical strain on his or her relationship with the patient.[31] For example, if a physician in a large group with a centralized fund orders an MRI to evaluate a young woman for multiple sclerosis, cost will not be a primary concern, because it is spread out over the group. If that same physician orders the MRI and the money comes out of his or her own capitated fund, it directly impacts that physician's income. The temptation to assign a heart murmur a benign status or to forego a cardiology consult is greater if every penny spent comes out of the physician's own pocket. Most conscientious physicians will resist this temptation, but it injects an unnecessary "ethical stress" into the clinical encounter, and may in some cases influence treatment decisions to the detriment of good patient care. Many HMOs now shy away from such direct capitation, and instead capitate physicians as a group.

CONSEQUENCES OF MANAGED CARE FINANCIAL INCENTIVES

What are the possible consequences of capitation and other financial inducements to physicians to control costs? The most widely discussed is the temptation to withhold needed services.[32] Whether this really happens is hard to prove, and has not been supported in the few studies that have examined the question.[33] However, anecdotes about harm to patients from undertreatment abound, and this issue remains a primary concern of those who study managed care.[34] It may also be that a disincentive arises to retain ill patients in one's health plan or patient panel, as they will tend to cost more than they (or their employers) pay into the plan. This could endanger the care of patients with complex chronic illnesses, such as AIDS.[35]

The beneficial impact of managed care incentives includes the reduction of wasteful treatments, less iatrogenic harm to patients by the avoidance of unnecessary tests and procedures, more emphasis on preventive care, the potential for better case management of very ill patients in an integrated setting,[36] and cost savings.[37] All of these benefits result in improvements in the quality of the care provided under managed care.[38] Although the degree of cost savings under managed care also has been contested,[39] this is the aspect of managed care that has propelled it to the forefront of health care delivery systems.

BALANCING THE INCENTIVE TO UNDERTREAT

So far, I have focused primarily on the financial relationships that are intended to influence physician behavior and to decrease health care costs. But physicians are influenced by nonfinancial considerations as well.[40] What kinds of incentives exist that may balance or buffer the temptation to limit treatment for the physician's own pecuniary benefit?

The strongest forces that balance the temptation to undertreat are the principles most physicians acquired in medical school.[41] The most important and pervasive principle is the professional duty to benefit, or at least not harm, their patients. Applying this principle in traditional FFS would counteract the temptation to overtreat. Under managed care, physicians will be less likely to withhold necessary treatments if their primary allegiance is to the patient's well-being.[42] Next in importance is the maintenance of the physician's professional and personal integrity, which again requires that they prevent harm to their patients. The approval of one's colleagues also exerts a strong effect on the behavior of many physicians, and is why peer review is such a powerful tool to change physician behavior. If the philosophy and practice of the physician group reflect the primacy of good patient care over all other considerations, it is less likely that patients will suffer under managed care.[43] Reinforcing these principles in medical school and residency will be an important factor in maintaining good patient care as practiced in the managed care setting.

Health systems have mechanisms for reinforcing the principle of beneficence and for maintaining high quality patient care, such as peer review and practice guidelines. These mechanisms, for example, give the physician feedback if he or she is not providing the quality for care that colleagues expect, or let a physician know, for example, if he or she is not ordering enough mammograms or vaccinations. The threat of malpractice is a reality in all treatment settings, and it can both promote overtreatment in FFS and deter undertreatment in managed care (see Table 3). State and federal regulations, and future legislation will also impact MCOs.[44] Finally, if health plan subscribers are educated and involved in their health care, they may be less likely to accept inadequate care, and more likely to understand the financial trade-offs involved in every health care decision.

Table 3. Forces Balancing the Negative Consequences of Managed Care Incentives.	
Principles of Practice	**External Approaches**
Desire to prevent harm from undertreatment (beneficence)	Treatment guidelines
Professionalism/self-respect (integrity)	Peer review
Desire for the respect of ones' peers	Fear of malpractice
	Patient/member involvement
	Regulation and legislation

THE ETHICAL HMO

Enumerating ethical principles and good practices is not enough to help us identify those organizations that are best-suited to promote the provision of health care in an atmosphere relatively untainted by financial conflicts of interest. Many authors have developed important and useful guidelines and principles for MCOs,[45] but I would like to summarize from the above discussion the structural features of health care organizations that nurture and reinforce the best principles of medical practice. MCO structure determines in large part the nature of the conflicts providers within it have to face, and it can also impact the quality of the care delivered.[46] For example, pre-approval admission requirements for hospitalization are a structural barrier to good patient care. A direct financial incentive to reduce hospital admissions is an ethical hurdle the physician must overcome to keep the patient's welfare foremost.

What would MCO look like were it structured to buffer or neutralize the incentives to undertreat patients and to maximize the incentives to provide quality medical care? What features should we look for in evaluating the degree of ethical stress a physician experiences in providing health care in different practice settings?

- The organization should be non-profit.[47] This removes shareholders and profit maximization as the bottom line, which theoretically puts less pressure on the physician to meet financial goals (as opposed to patient outcome goals).

- To remove the cash register from the examination room, physicians should be salaried.[48] Divorcing the individual patient encounter from the physician's immediate income helps to focus the encounter on meeting the patient's needs, and frees the physician to practice according to his or her professional principles. Group model and staff model HMOs both meet this ideal.

- Sharing the risk of capitation across a large group of physicians dilutes the temptation to cut corners inappropriately.[49] The manner in which capitated funds are distributed varies and influences the degree of conflict of interest the physician experiences. Direct or individual capitation and linking financial incentives directly to cost-containment targets should be avoided.

- Clinical practice should be managed by physicians. Physicians should be heavily involved with utilization review, quality management, and the development and implementation of practice guidelines. Utilization review should not serve as a barrier to providing health care services.

- The patients or members of the MCO should have a role in the operations of the organization, at a number of levels.[50] First, subscribers should receive full disclosure from the health plan about any incentives to limit treatment and any restrictions on coverage. Second, MCOs need to find a mechanism to include health plan members in discussions of benefit coverage and conflict resolution procedures. Third, community members should be involved in the ethics committees of managed care hospitals and in the organizational ethics committees of health plans, where these committees exist.[51] Fourth, vigorous efforts at patient/member health education should be fundamental, both to improve the health of members and to improve their understanding of the financial trade-offs involved in treatment and benefit decisions. An educated member may be more likely to challenge unfair limits to treatment.

CONCLUSION

Managed care is not one entity, it is a broad umbrella that includes a variety of health care delivery structures, relationships with physicians and physician incentives. While all managed care forms face the challenge of avoiding undertreatment, some are more challenged than others. Whether an MCO minimizes conflicts of interest for physicians depends on the way it is organized and financed, the degree of physician involvement in managing patient care quality, and the nature of the incentives used to control costs. The form of managed care which currently works best to prevent undertreatment is one that is nonprofit and has a large salaried physician group that manages the clinical aspects of the provision of health care services.

Having drawn these distinctions, it is clear that managed care as a subject of study is a rapidly moving target. Non-profit HMOs themselves are sorely challenged to compete with the for-profit entities.[52] All are taking measures to cut costs, and, in many instances, are adopting the methods of the for-profit HMOs.[53] If this trend continues, it is possible that the distinction between for-profit and nonprofit MCOs will blur. Moreover, for-profit organizations are rearranging themselves into new and unique forms at a rapid rate.[54] Thus, as these new structures evolve, we must encourage the growth of those that foster the highest quality of patient care and physician satisfaction.

ACKNOWLEDGMENT

I thank the following people for their generous contribution of ideas and comments: Robert Klein, M.D.; William Andereck, M.D.; Jim Rose; Francis J. Crosson, M.D.; Robert Erickson; Lawrence Schneiderman, M.D.; Bruce Merl, M.D.; Cecilia Runkle, Ph.D.; Art Rosenfeld, J.D.; and Bernard Lo, M.D.

This article is based on a presentation given at "Managed Care Systems: Emerging Health Issues from an Ethics Perspective," sponsored by the Allina Foundation and the American Society of Law, Medicine & Ethics, Minneapolis, Minnesota, June 1995.
20.

KEY IDEAS FROM THIS ARTICLE:

- Managed care is not one entity; it is a broad umbrella that includes a variety of structures, relationships with physicians, and physician incentives. While all managed care forms face the challenge of avoiding undertreatment, some are more challenged than others.

- There are three crucial distinctions to be made among MCOs: profit status, relationship of physicians to the organization, and the nature of the capitation arrangements.

Profit status:

- The most important distinction to be made among MCOs is their profit status.

- The administrative costs (marketing, cash reserves, dividends to share-holders, etc.) of for-profit MCOs tends to be much higher than that of not-for-profit MCOs.

- It stands to reason that physicians in an MCO that has both less to spend on patient care and stockholders to please will be under more pressure to cut corners.

Relationship of Physicians to the Organization:

- Experience to date indicates that when control over the clinical aspects of practice rests with nonphysician administrators, the quality of patient care and physician morale plummets.

- When managed and implemented by physicians, utilization review can both promote better patient care and save money.

- When physicians are involved in developing practice guidelines, such guidelines serve as a useful extension of peer review and help maintain a high quality of care. Such physician involvement helps avoid using such guidelines as standards to measure, reward, and punish physician behavior.

Incentives:

- While capitation forms the core financial process in MCOs, the more individualized the capitation arrangement is in relation to the physician, the greater the ethical strain on his or her relationship with the patient.

- The beneficial impact of financial incentives includes: reduction of waste, less iatrogenic harm, more emphasis on preventive care, potential for better case management of the very ill, and cost savings.

- Peer review has a powerful impact on physician behavior, and if the philosophy and practice of the physician group reflect the primacy of good patient care over all other considerations, it is less likely that patients will suffer under managed care.

The ethical HMO:

Since MCO structure determines in large part the nature of the conflicts providers will have to face, and also impacts the quality of the care delivered, what structural elements matter?

- The organization should be non-profit.

- Physicians should be salaried.

- Capitation risk should be shared across large groups of physicians to dilute the temptation to cut corners.

- Physicians should be heavily involved with utilization review quality management, and the development and implementation of practice guidelines.

- Patients should be vitally involved on many levels:
    - full disclosure to subscribers about incentives and limitations of treatment;
    - participation in determining benefit coverage and conflict resolution;
    - membership on ethics committees;
    - vigorous patient/member education about the nature of managed care.

A SUGGESTED PROCESS FOR REFLECTING ON THIS ARTICLE:

(see pages 234-254 for other processes that might better fit your specific goals and objectives).

Issue	I personally agree: 1-5, 5=high	Consensus in our organization	Consensus in professional discussion
MCO structure determines in large part the nature of the conflicts providers will have to face, and also impacts the quality of the care delivered.			
The organization should be non-profit.			
Physicians should be salaried.			
Captitation risk should be shared across large groups of physicians to dilute the temptation to cut corners.			
Physicians should be heavily involved with utilization review quality management, and the development and implementation of practice guidelines.			
Patients should be vitally involved – e.g., full disclosure to subscribers about incentives and limitations of treatment.			
Patients should be vitally involved – e.g., participation in determining benefit coverage and conflict resolution.			
Patients should be vitally involved – e.g., membership on ethics committees.			
Patients should be vitally involved – e.g., vigorous patient/member education about the nature of managed care.			

IN LIGHT OF OUR DISCUSSION:

- as (executive committee, ethics committee, etc.), what are some next steps that we should take?

- as (hospital, home health agency, etc.), what are some next steps that we should take?

- what systems and structures call for special attention in order to improve the situation?

ENDNOTES

1. Marc A. Rodwin, *Medicine, Money & Morals: Physicians' Conflicts of Interest* (New York: Oxford, 1993): at 17; John Fletcher and Carolyn Engelhard, "Ethical Issues in Managed Care," *Virginia Medicine Quarterly,* 122, no. 3 (1995): 162-67; Michael Quint, "Health Plans Force Changes in the Way Doctors Are Paid," *New York Times,* Feb. 9, 1995, at Al; Arnold S. Relman, "Medical Practice Under the Clinton Reforms – Avoiding Domination by Business," *N. Engl. J. Med.,* 329 (1993): 1574-76; and Mike Mitka, "HMOs See Steady Growth, Some Market Shifts," *American Medical News,* May 1, 1995, at 9.

2. Milt Freudenheim, "Medicare, Jot This Down: Employers Offer Valuable Lessons on Saving Money with Managed Care," *New York Times,* May 31, 1995, at Cl; Julie Johnson, "Medicare's Bumpy Ride into Private Sector," *American Medical News,* June 12, 1995, at 1; Adam Clymer, "An Accidental Overhaul: Major Revamping of Health Care System Could be Byproduct of Steep Budget Cuts," *New York Times,* June 26, 1995, at Al; and Milt Freudenheim, "Corporations Step up Efforts to Get Retirees into H.M.O.'s," *New York Times,* June 13, 1995, at C1.

3. Arnold S. Relman, "The Impact of Market Forces on the Physician-Patient Relationship," *Journal of the Royal Society of Medicine,* 87 (supp. 22) (1994): 22 -25; Arnold S. Relman, "Medical Insurance and Health: What about Managed Care?," *N. Engl. J. Med.,* 331 (1994): 471-72; and Edmund Pellegrino, "Ethics," *JAMA,* 271 (1994): 1668-70.

4. Julie Johnsson, "Megamerger of Two Public Plans Spurs New Interest in Stock Offering," *American Medical News,* Apr. 24, 1995, at 1; and Milt Freudenheim, "Penny-Pinching H.M.O.'s Showed Their Generosity in Executive Paychecks," *New York Times,* Apr. 11, 1995, at Cl.

5. Cal. Code Non-Profit Corp., §§5130-B (West 1980).

6. See Freudenheim, *supra* note 4; and Marc Rodwin, "Conflicts in Managed Care," *N. Engl. J. Med.,* 332 (1995): 604-07.

7. Steve Thompson and Zabrae Valentine, "The Profiteering of HMOs," *California Physician,* July 1994, at 28-32, based on a California Department of Corporations report for 1992.

8. Alameda-Contra Costa Medical Association, "Latest CMA Study Shows Rise in HMO Costs and Profits," *ACCMA Bulletin,* Feb. 1995, at 14; and Milt Freudenheim, "A Bitter Pill for the HMO's," *New York Times,* Apr. 28, 1995, at Cl.

9. See Freudenheim, *supra* note 6; and Michael Hiltzik and David Olmos, "Are Executives at HMOs Paid Too Much Money?," *Los Angeles Times,* Aug. 30, 1995, at A13.

10. See Fletcher and Engelhard, *supra* note 1.

11. John M. Eisenberg, "Economics," *JAMA,* 273 (1995): 1670-71.

12. Alan Hillman, "Financial Incentives for Physicians in HMOs: Is There a Conflict of Interest?," *N. Engl. J. Med.,* 317 (1987): 1743-48; see Rodwin, *supra* note 1, at 152 -56.

13. Linda Prager, "State Licensing Boards Consider Curbing Financial Incentives," *American Medical News,* Oct. 16, 1995, at 1, 74.

14. Ezekiel Emanuel and Nancy N. Dubler, "Preserving the Physician-Patient Relationship in the Era of Managed Care," *JAMA, 273* (1995): 323-29; see Rodwin, *supra* note 1, at 98.

15. Lisa Krieger, "Family Doctors are Disappearing," San *Francisco Examiner,* June 18, 1995, at A1.

16. David Olmos, "Some Doctors Head to Idaho, a State Without Managed Care," *Los Angeles Times,* Aug. 29, 1995, at A11.

17. Seymour Herschberg, "Potential Conflicts of Interest in the Delivery of Medical Services: An Analysis of the Situation and a Proposal," *Quality Assurance and Utilization Review,* 7 (1992): 54-58.

18. Budd Shenkin, "The Independent Practice Association in Theory and Practice," *JAMA,* 273 (1995): 1937-42.

19. Emily Friedman, "Changing the System: Implications for Physicians," *JAMA,* 269 (1993): 2437-42.

20. Council on Ethical and Judicial Affairs, American Medical Association, "Ethical Issues in Managed Care," *JAMA,* 273 (1995): 330-35.

21. See Rodwin, *supra* note 1, at 138-44.

22. See Relman, *supra* note 1; and Vincent Cangello, "The Real Issue," *ACCMA Bulletin,* Jan. 1995, at 18.

23. Michael Hiltzik, "Emergency Rooms, HMOs Clash over Treatments and Payments," *Los Angeles Times,* Aug. 30, at A12.

24. William Phillips, letter: "Hassle Hypertension: A Risk of Managed Care," *JAMA,* 274 (1995): 795-96.

25. See Rodwin, *supra* note 1, at 135.

26. One study of IPAs and physician groups with capitated contracts shows that physicians tend to employ the same type of barriers to care, such as pre-authorization requirements, as health plans,. The study did not include the largest group practice HMO in California, Kaiser Permanente, which does not use pre-authorization requirements to control costs. Eve Kerr et al., "Managed Care and Capitation in California: How Do Physicians at Financial Risk Control Their Own Utilization?," *Annals of Internal Medicine,* 123 (1995): 500-04.

27. Francis J. Crosson, "Why Outcomes Measurement Must be the Basis for the Development of Clinical Guidelines," *Managed Care Quarterly,* 3, no. 2 (1995): 6-11; David Eddy, "Broadening the Responsibilities of Practitioners: The Team Approach," *JAMA,* 268 (1993): 1849-55; and Les Zendle, "Controlling Costs:The Case of Kaiser," *JAMA,* 274 (1995): 1135.

28. See Friedman, *supra* note 19.

29. See Crosson, *supra* note 27.

30. Alan Hillman, "Health Maintenance Organizations, Financial Incentives, and Physicians' Judgments," *Annals of Internal Medicine,* 112 (1990): 891-93.

31. Rodwin, *supra* note 1, at 139-41.

32. Nancy S. Jecker, "Managed Competition and Managed Care," *Clinics in Geriatric Medicine, 10* (1994): 527-40; see Emanuel and Dubler, *supra* note 14; and Council on Ethical and Judicial Affairs, *supra* note 20.

33. Dolores Clement et al., "Access and Outcomes for Elderly Patients Enrolled in Managed Care," *JAMA,* 271 (1994): 1487-92.

34. See Council on Ethical and Judicial Affairs, *supra* note 20; Daniel Sulmasy, "Managed Care and Managed Death," *Archives of Internal Medicine,* 155 (1995): 133-36; and Michael Hiltzik and David Olmos, "A Mixed Diagnosis for HMO's," *Los Angeles Times,* Aug. 27, 1995, at A1.

35. Julius Richmond, "The Health Care Mess," *JAMA,* 273 (1995): 69-71.

36. Steven Miles, "End-of-Life Treatment in Managed Care: The Potential and the Peril," *Western Journal of Medicine,* 163 (1995): 302-05.

37. See Eisenberg, *supra* note 11; and "Study: Managed Care Lowers Hospital Costs, Improves Quality," *American Medical News,* June 19, 1995, at 6.

38. Joan Meisel, *Quality of Care in HMOs: A Review of the Literature* (Sacramento: CAHMO, Sept. 1994); California Cooperative HEDIS Reporting Initiative, *Report on Quality of Care Measures* (San Francisco: CCHRI, Feb. 1995); and National Committee for Quality Assurance, *Report Card Pilot Project Technical Report* (New York: NCQA, 1994).

39. Janice Somerville, "CMA Study: High HMO Administrative Costs for Medicaid," *American Medical News,* May 15, 1995, at 12.

40. See Hillman, *supra* note 12.

41. Woodstock Theological Center, *Ethical Considerations in the Business Aspects of Health Care* (Washington, D.C.: Georgetown University Press, 1995): at 9-14.

42. *Id.* at 20-22.

43. Board of Directors of Kaiser Foundation Hospitals and Kaiser Foundation Health Plan, "Principles of Responsibility" (1984): in-house circular.

44. Forces external to managed care are exerting a growing pressure against under-treatment. For example, the 1990 Medicare amendment restricts prepaid plans contracting with the Health Care Financing Administration from creating an "incentive plan as an inducement to reduce or limit medically necessary services to a specific individual." See Medicare law in 42 U.S.C. §§1395mm(i)(8)(A) (1990). Legislation pending in several states would put limits on the type of cost-control measures that MCOs can employ. See Eugene Ogrod, "The Many Faces of Managed Care," *California Physician,* Aug. 1995, at 10; and Julie Johnsson, "State Laws on Managed Care Spur New Battles," *American Medical News,* July 24, 1995, at 3, 51.

45. Joan D. Biblo et al., *Ethical Issues in Managed Care: Guidelines for Clinicians and Recommendations to Accrediting Organizations* (Kansas City: Midwest Bioethics Center, 1995); Susan M. Wolf, "Health Care Reform and the Future of Physician Ethics," *Hastings Center Report,* 24, no. 2 (1994): 28-41; see Council on Ethical and Judicial Affairs, *supra* note 20; and H. Tristram Engelhardt and Michael A. Rie, "Morality for Medical-Industrial Complex: A Code of Ethics for the Mass Marketing of Health Care," *N. Engl. J. Med.,* 319 (1988): 1086-89.

46. Donald Barr, "The Effects of Organizational Structure on Primary Care Outcomes under Managed Care," *Annals of Internal Medicine,* 122 (1995): 353-59.

47. See Relman, *supra* note 1. Marcia Angell, "The Beginning of Health Care Reform: The Clinton Plan," *N. Engl. J. Med.,* 329 (1993): 1569-70; and Cardinal Joseph Bernadin, "Making the Case for Not-for-Profit Healthcare," speech by Cardinal Joseph Bernadin, Harvard Business School Club of Chicago, Jan. 12, 1995.

48. See Rodwin, *supra* note 1, at 136.

49. See Council on Ethical and Judicial Affairs, *supra* note 20.

50. Ezekiel Emanuel, "Managed Competition and the Patient-Physician Relationship," *N. Engl. J. Med., 329* (1993): 879-82.

51. Jonathan Harding, "The Role of Organizational Ethics Committees," *Physician Executive,* 20, no. 2 (1994): 19-24; see Emanuel and Dubler, *supra* note 14.

52. David Azevedo, "Can the World's Largest Integrated Health System Learn to Feel Small?," *Medical Economics*, 72, no. 2 (1995): 82-103.

53. David Azevedo, "What You Can Bargain for When HMO's Compete," *Business & Health,* June (1995): 44-56.

54. Michael Quint, "Merger to Create Largest Company for Health Plans," *New York Times,* June 27, 1995, at Al.

CHAPTER 11

THE ETHICS OF INCENTIVES IN MANAGED CARE

E. Haavi Morriem, Ph.D.

INTRODUCTION

Ethical issues can be found in managed care on both a policy level and a clinical level. On the policy level, managed care organizations (MCOs) face questions of justice: as they determine what kinds of care to provide for whom, and when, they must balance the needs of individual enrollees against those of the larger group. MCOs must set limits on facilities, for instance, from hospital beds and clinic offices to medical staff. And new technologies, such as autologous bone marrow transplant for breast cancer, offer uncertain potential to save lives at very high cost. Each individual subscriber has a legitimate claim to the care that he needs, yet MCOs must guard against excessive expenditures that could threaten their fiscal (vi)ability to serve the other subscribers with the care to which they are morally and contractually entitled.

MCOs manage resources, not just by policies governing facilities and costly new technologies, but also by bringing cost-consciousness to the delivery of ordinary care. These devices create ethical issues on the clinical level. Utilization review (UR) can limit physicians' clinical autonomy. If the guideline does not fit a patient's needs, the physician faces *conflicts of obligation,* pitting his contractual duty to honor the MCO's rules against his fiduciary obligation to serve each patient's best interests. Incentive systems, on the other hand, leave physicians considerably freer to exercise their clinical judgment, but only by creating *conflicts of interest* that pit their own interests against their patients.[1]

This article argues that these ethical problems are partly the product of an economic structure that brings the economic incentives of physicians into harmony with those of the MCO, while leaving patients under a completely different set of incentives, and thereby expectations. Whereas providers are rewarded for delivering a conservative level of care, patients' economic insulation encourages them to ignore costs and to demand a high level of care as their entitlement. The article then proposes that if MCOs rewarded patients for using the system conservatively, patients would have more reason to consider which care is worthwhile, and physicians' incentives could be shifted toward promoting quality of care. Changing patients' economic incentives will not resolve all the moral issues of managed care, but it can considerably ease policy conflicts between patients and MCOs, and reduce physicians' clinical conflicts of interest and conflicts of obligation.

HISTORICAL PERSPECTIVE

Until recently, modern healthcare financing was largely retrospective, fee-for-service and generous. Insurers reimbursed largely according to whatever fees providers said they customarily charged, and rarely challenged medical (i.e., spending) decisions. Insurers passed on cost increases to businesses, that in turn reaped tax write-offs. Providers were economically insulated, knowing that they would be paid for virtually any service rendered (the more services the better), and most patients were likewise insulated from costs, either by first-dollar coverage through the workplace or by a cost-shifting in which those who could not pay were subsidized by those who could.[2]

The system was, in essence, an Artesian Well of Money. Virtually no one had much reason to worry about the cost of care. And so long as money was no object, certain values prevailed. Among them:

- potentially beneficial care should never be denied on account of mere money;

- an individual's (in)ability to pay is irrelevant to the kind and level of care he should receive;

- physicians should never compromise their patients' care in order to save money, except perhaps where the patient is paying (thus presuming that insurance money is not ultimately patients' money);

- other things being equal, it is generally better to intervene too much than too little (high-tech is better than low-tech is better than no-tech).[3]

Even the legal system has expected physicians to provide all patients with an essentially identical and rather lavish standard of care – sometimes including costly technologies – regardless of the patient's ability to pay, and regardless of who owns the technologies or pays for their use. In this sense, the legal system has expected physicians virtually to commandeer other people's money and property for their patients' use.[4]

These Artesian values, alongside the inflationary reimbursement system and other factors, such as the rise of high technology and the aging of the population, sent health care costs into the upward spiral that governments and businesses are now trying so frantically to stem. Cost containment initially focused on controls, such as wage/price freezes and regulatory limits on construction and capital acquisition.[5] However, as controls failed, it became evident that providers' Artesian incentives had to be changed.

In 1973 Congress permitted health maintenance organizations (HMOs) to reverse almost completely the providers' traditional incentives to maximize care. Under the necessity to provide all subscribers' care within a fixed annual budget, HMO physicians and hospitals questioned the necessity of many standard forms of care, including the facile use of hospitalization and aggressive technology, and focused instead on keeping patients healthy and delivering only necessary interventions in appropriate settings. HMOs were not just permitted, but expected to ensure physicians' cost-consciousness with appropriate incentives.[6]

Even the fee-for-service sector saw incentives change. In 1982, Congress established Diagnosis-Related Group (DRG) reimbursement, setting a fixed fee for each hospital admission of Medicare patients. Instead of reaping revenue by keeping patients longer and providing more services, hospitals now could only profit by limiting length of stay and intensity of care.

Significantly, DRGs directly affected only hospitals, leaving physicians under Artesian incentives. Clashes were inevitable as hospitals, needing to "do less" confronted physicians, accustomed to "do more," so hospitals sought to bring physicians under the new incentives. Nasty memos from annoyed administrators eventually gave way to more concrete tactics, such as publishing physicians' spending patterns at staff meetings in hopes of using peer pressure and embarrassment to change old habits.[7] More recently, a far more powerful tool has emerged: economic credentialing, the denial or revocation of staff privileges for high-spenders.[8]

The impetus toward conservative care has become even stronger as businesses and governments require providers to compete with each other to offer the best healthcare packages at the lowest prices. All providers, whether physicians, hospitals or MCOs, are beginning to realize they must limit costs. After all, every medical decision is a spending decision. Particularly in the financially more closed systems of managed care, what is spent on one patient is not available for other patients or purposes. And so the language of "aligning" incentives now predominates.

If patients and treatments are to be effectively "managed," the principal instruments of medical practice, namely physicians, must operate under the same constraints. Hence, we are witnessing the creation and development of corporate entities and financial arrangements meant to bring physicians *into concert* with payors, managed care organizations and hospitals. If fully *aligned,* this trio of payors, providers (doctors and hospitals), and managed care organizations will be organized *cooperatively* and positioned to produce the change necessary to rewrite, even revolutionize American medicine.[9]

Note in this description that patients are not listed among the financial players. They remain in the Artesian Well, excluded from the new economic incentives. In another example of alignment language, Sulmasy notes that "[w]hat is envisioned under managed competition is thus a three-layered system. The government manages HMOs, HMOs manage physicians, and physicians manage patients. All three would have strong incentives to spend less on health care." As above, although the passage identifies four parties – government, HMOs, physicians and patients – only three are contemplated as players in managing care.

Admittedly, patients' economic insulation is beginning to erode. Rather few people with indemnity insurance still enjoy first-dollar coverage, while many others face increased cost-sharing. But the effect is limited. Copayments are still fairly small for most patients; many people have "gap" insurance to cover such copays; many others expect their physicians to waive copays, or they simply refuse to pay. Costs are rarely discussed at the time treatment decisions are made. More important for this discussion, patients in MCOs remain especially insulated from the economic consequences of their healthcare decisions. Typically, copayments are extremely modest, a few dollars for a physician visit or prescription.

The justifications for continuing patients' economic insulation vary: it is feared that any economic incentives should create financial obstacles to needed care, or that patients might make medically foolish decisions in order to save money, or that patients are incapable of understanding economic factors enough to take reasonable account of them in making decisions (even though they are entitled through the principle of informed consent to make vastly more complicated medical decisions). The defects in these rationales are addressed elsewhere.[11] Instead, this article focuses on the ways in which this profound discrepancy between providers' and patients' incentives creates serious ethical problems and how, even with in MCOs, bringing patients' incentives into alignment with providers' can ameliorate those problems significantly.

DIVERGING INCENTIVES: FORMULA FOR TROUBLE

The consequences of these sharply divergent incentives are serious. To begin with, patients with an Artesian mentality often believe that health care is free, that they have an unlimited right to the best medical care, spare no expenses.[12] If consulted about what providers or treatments their health plan should offer, they may well answer "everything."[13]

Second, and more importantly, because patients remain insulated and naive about the economics of care, their preferences about their health plans are largely disregarded. Patients are steadily losing control. Businesses that provide health coverage commonly limit employees' health plan choices to a few options that suit their own, not necessarily the employees' best interests. Of businesses that do provide healthcare insurance, about 84% provide only one option.[14] Many of the rest provide only two choices. After all, it is employers who directly pay for the plans, and it is they who enjoy the savings of less-expensive plans.

In turn, the health plans choose their physicians, not just on the basis of quality but also for their willingness to contain costs. Those who don't fit with the MCO's financial objectives are likely to be "deselected" (fired). And in the next turn, plans and their physicians limit the available diagnostic and treatment options. In sum: employers choose the plans, the plans choose the providers, and the plans with their providers choose the treatment options. The patient is largely left out, and often has just one choice: take it or leave it.

The combination is a dangerous, vicious cycle. The same economic insulation that renders patients too naive to use resources prudently – and, therefore, not fit to participate in resource decisions – gives them every Artesian reason to demand the best of everything. They directly pay little or nothing for their care, and have little or no reward for frugality. Accordingly, patients lose plan, provider and treatment choices, while employers, plans and physicians pocket the savings.

This combination of patients' high expectations and lack of control can translate into substantial pressures on physicians. Physicians still largely control healthcare resources through their license to practice medicine and their power of prescription. But patients can still exert demands, sometimes by appealing to the physician's ethic of fidelity, and sometimes by threatening to use their lone-remaining weapon of control: the lawsuit.[15] As a result, physicians are caught systematically, sometimes hopelessly, between the conflicting incentives of patients and health plans. Patients insist "do more," while MCOs command them "do less."

The inevitable result is adversarial. Patients may become adversaries of physicians who refuse to prescribe a requested antibiotic or to authorize a referral for consultation. They may feel that their physician is a stranger who neither knows them nor cares about them.[16] Alternatively, physicians and patients together may be adversaries of the MCO. Where a physician wants to "do more," he can adeptly game the system to extract extra resources.[17]

Reciprocally, MCOs may become adversaries of patients and physicians. In California, a number of physicians believed they were being deselected from MCOs after protesting UR denials on their patients' behalf. In response, a new statute was legislated to protect physicians who can show they were deselected as retaliation for their patient advocacy.[18]

Attempting to minimize such controversy and gaming, many MCOs take care not to disclose their cost constraints to patients, particularly incentive arrangements. If patients do not know that physicians increase their outcome by decreasing patients' care, it is thought they may be less suspicious when they do not receive the level of medical care they expected. Indeed, some MCOs actually have so-called "gag clauses," forbidding physicians to disclose to patients any information that might reflect poorly on the MCO. One "large managed care plan, said to represent about 85% of Cincinnati physicians, recently gagged its participating physicians, ruling that they 'shall take no action nor make any communication which undermines or could undermine the confidence of enrollees, potential enrollees, their employees, plan sponsors, or the public in [the plan] or in the quality of care which [its] members receive.' "[19] Such secrecy is yet another adversarial element as MCOs presume patients cannot be trusted with information about the health plan they have bought.

RESOLUTION: BRINGING PATIENTS INTO INCENTIVES

To recap: patients' economic insulation, and the wide disparity of incentives between patients and providers, fuels two of the most prominent ethical problems in managed care. At the policy level, patients are excluded from important resource decisions that profoundly affect them and, at the clinical level, physicians are placed in systematic conflicts of interest that threaten traditional obligations of fidelity. If this is so, then perhaps those problems might be reduced, at the policy level, by including patients in resource decisions and, at the clinical level, by bringing them into the economic incentives that guide physicians and MCOs.

Both levels would be important. At the lower level, clinical incentives could involve patients better in decisions about the more modestly priced, routine kinds of care – the minor expenses that other kinds of insurance do not cover at all. Under the sort of incentives to be proposed below, most people would be rewarded for prudent resource use. About 85% of Americans spend less than $3000 a year on medical care; and 73% less than $500.[20]

On the other hand, most of the money spent on health care is for a relatively few patients with severe acute injuries and illnesses and costly chronic conditions. Here there is rather little room for financial incentives, since the costs run so high. Rather, plans need prudent resource policies to govern what sorts of care should be provided for whom. Here, too, patients should be involved in resource planning. It is they whose lives are most intimately affected and, ultimately, it is they who are paying the bills.

1. Policy level

The first policy-level change should be for MCOs to inform patients about their resource policies. This information would encompass physicians' incentive systems and other utilization controls, such as therapeutic substitution requirements.[21] Arguably, the commonplace practice of keeping such arrangements secret is ethically and legally wrong. And practically speaking, it is probably not even possible much longer.

Morally and legally, physicians already have duties to disclose incentive schemes to patients. This is because physicians are fiduciaries, and fiduciaries have clear legal and ethical obligations to promote their beneficiaries' interests, even above their own. They also must disclose any conflicts of interest that might encourage them to place their own interests above their patients'. Because MCO incentive systems create conflicts of interest by paying physicians more money to deliver less care, physicians are obligated to disclose them.[22]

Arguably, if physicians must disclose these incentives, so should the MCO that created them.[23] Admittedly, there is no technical requirement to do so, even though HMOs must disclose certain kinds of information, such as the scope and limits of benefits packages and procedures for appealing denials of benefits.[24] However, MCOs can also be regarded as fiduciaries, both as financial insurers and as providers of care.[25] As such they, too, would owe common-law duties of disclosure and the utmost deference to the interests of subscribers.[26] Arguments based on contract law may also apply. If HMOs, as drafters of their contracts with subscribers, have not clearly specified limits on services, or in their advertisements have exaggerated the level of care they deliver, they may be at fault for fraud, breach of contract or other civil wrongs.[27]

Practically speaking, concealment is hardly feasible much longer. Once a physician makes the necessary disclosure, the MCO's question whether to disclose it is moot. For another thing, a rising tide of lawsuits cites MCOs' failure to disclose incentive arrangements among their allegations.[26] As these suits inflame the media, increasing numbers of MCO subscribers may suspect that their care, too, is constrained by similar incentive arrangements.

Adequate disclosures by MCOs of their incentive systems and resource limits need not be prohibitively awkward. First, as already noted, many people already knows about them through sensational lawsuits and news stories. Second, physicians and MCOs can explain that all health care financiers and providers must contain costs, and that virtually all of them use the same basic approaches – UR and incentives. In other words: competing plans do the same thing – they just aren't telling. The provider that discloses its resource policies forthrightly may win trust from people otherwise cynical about the healthcare industry. Third, MCOs can show that careful resource use serves, rather than harms subscribers' interests. All members' care comes from a finite sum of money, and if the MCO gives in to the other subscribers' excessive demands, there will be less money left for this individual.

Beyond disclosures, the MCO should actively involve subscribers in important policy decisions. Should patients with myocardial infarction receive costly TPA, which may (or may not) yield slightly improved survival, rather than much cheaper streptokinase? Should the plan pay for endless intensive care of patients in a persistent vegetative state? Should the plan cover costly but promising new treatments, whose medical value is not scientifically documented, such as bone marrow transplant for breast cancer?

Policies governing what levels of care an MCO covers should at least be influenced, even if not determined, by those who are most affected by them and who ultimately pay for them, namely patients. Federally qualified HMOs were originally required to have policy boards, with at least one-third of their members subscribers. Although that requirement has largely disappeared, most states required some subscriber participation in the health plan's policy decisions.[29] Some HMOs have long traditions of involving subscribers.[30] This element of managed care needs to be reinvigorated.

2. Clinical level

Unfortunately, such policy participation probably will not work well until the major problem – the incentive discrepancy – is resolved. So long as patients experience virtually no economic consequences of their medical spending decisions, it remains easy to expect unlimited benefits. So policy preferences may simply amount to a demand for the best, spare no expense.[31] This may be particularly true in MCOs, where cost-sharing is minimal.

At the same time, financial consequences must not represent barriers to care. After all, a centerpiece of managed care is assured access to care without financial impediment. Thus, the goal must be to reward patients for prudence without impeding needed care.

There are many ways to construct such a system, but only one will be outlined here. Analogous to a Medical-Savings Account,[32] each subscriber might begin each year with a certain number of "HMO-dollars" or points. Each time the subscriber receives medical care, points could be deducted, perhaps on a standard per-service format, or maybe proportionate to the intensity (cost) of the actual services delivered. To encourage preventive care, patients might earn extra points for seeking immunizations, mammograms or the like. Those with chronic illnesses might likewise be awarded points for securing important follow-up care. Patients wanting interventions exceeding the MCO's guidelines, such as a CT scan for ordinary tension headaches, or a costly drug not on the formulary, might "purchase" it by spending points.

Patients would still, of course, retain complete access to care. The points serve strictly as a reward for prudence, not a barrier requiring cash in order to secure care. The incentives are also indirect in that, unlike the copays and deductibles that many people now face, points are not pitted against current expenditures – one does not weigh health care directly against food at the time one decides whether to seek care.

At the end of each year, points might be redeemed for cash, or rolled over into the next year's account, or perhaps used toward in-kind rewards, such as health club memberships or even ordinary household goods. There are many ways to work out the details. The important feature is that conservative use of health services is directly, personally rewarded without creating financial barriers to care. All essential care is still completely covered. Although of course some patients with the most serious chronic or acute illnesses might end the year with little or no rebate, they can enjoy what is for them the best prize of all: greater access to the health services, as healthier patients opt for fewer unnecessary services and leave facilities and physicians more available to meet this group's more serious needs.

ADVANTAGES OF BRINGING PATIENTS INTO THE FINANCIAL INCENTIVES

There are many reasons why it is morally desirable to bring patients into alignment with providers' financial incentives. First, it respects patients as competent adults. Principles of autonomy and informed consent have long held that patients are entitled to determine what will happen to their own bodies. In the medical context, this means that the competent patient is entitled to accept or reject whatever interventions a physician offers, even for reasons that others might deem foolish or frivolous. It would be odd indeed to hold that, although a person is entitled to decide whether to refuse a life-saving blood transfusion, or to undergo a risky experimental treatment, he will not be permitted to decide how to spend his own money, on the ground that he might make a mistake, or that he might forego (what someone else has decided is) necessary care.

And it is his own money. Although the U.S. health care system has remarkably preserved the illusion that Someone Else, not the patient, pays for care, it is time to dispel the myth. Patients pay directly through out-of pocket cost-sharing, they pay as employees through foregone wages, other benefits, or even jobs, as taxpayers through higher taxes, and as consumers through higher prices.

Second, returning a measure of economic accountability to patients is probably the only way that they can regain a measure of control over their medical choices. So long as others, such as employers or MCOs, incur the direct costs and savings of medical resource use, they must and inevitably will control their costs – and thereby patients' care. Reciprocally, so long as patients are shielded from the economic consequences of their medical decisions, they have neither reason nor opportunity to consider which care is really worth its cost.[33] Hence, their preferences are likely to be regarded as economically and medically naive demands, and they will not be permitted to participate in important resource decisions. Their health plans, providers and treatments will be chosen by others – take it or leave it. Under an incentive system, however, the more that patients have reason to ask, "Do we really need this?" and "Can we safely watch and wait?" the less will outsiders need to. Only then are patients likely to be awarded greater control.[34]

A third advantage of bringing patients into financial incentives is its potential for restoring trust within the physician-patient relationship. The current system controls costs either by dictating, from the outside, what physicians can and cannot do or by placing physicians under incentives. Either the physician is helpless, as others forbid him to do what the patient requests, or he is in a personal conflict of interest.

If patients had reason and reward for considering costs more carefully, there would be less need for outsiders to decide which care is worth its cost, and thereby less need for intrusive and costly UR, and less gaming of the system. Indeed, the very concept of "managed" care presupposes that some third party must manage the economics of health care, on the assumption that physicians and patients cannot manage on their own.

Reciprocally, when the patient has a stake in the costs as well as the outcome of care, there is less need to incentivize the physician. At that point, the physician who explains that an intervention is unnecessary or unduly costly is no longer the enemy guarding a third party's resources. He is an ally, helping the patient to look out for his own larger interests, financial as well as medical. Patients do, after all, have lives outside the medical system, and can have priorities they consider more important than buying medical products and services. Such a physician will be in a powerful position to help patients, once the latter are under financial incentives, to avoid unwise medical decisions for the sake of short-term rewards. Probably the ideal incentive structure would reward physicians for quality of care, while rewarding patients for prudent cost-consciousness.

Finally, some other practical advantages might be anticipated. When patients have money as well as health interests at stake, even in minor healthcare decisions, they may be more interested to hear information and make choices carefully, thereby becoming more responsible for decisions and their outcomes. Where patients are more responsible, evidence indicates that they tend to be more satisfied with their care (even with adverse outcomes) and less apt to be litigious.[35]

In the final analysis, it is difficult to justify keeping patients insulated and isolated. If they are treated more as responsible adults, accountable for their decisions, with real economic consequences that nevertheless do not impede access to care, there may be considerably less adversity and mistrust in a relationship that should be, above all, a healing experience.

KEY IDEAS IN THIS ARTICLE:

- Until recently our health care system provided an Artesian Well of money which fostered values such as: potentially beneficial care should never be denied because of money; inability to pay should be irrelevant; physicians should never compromise care to save money; other things being equal, it is better to do too much than too little.

- In 1973 Congress permitted health maintenance organizations (HMOs) to reverse almost completely the providers' traditional incentives to maximize care.

- In 1982 Congress established DRGs, directly affecting only hospitals, leaving physicians under Artesian incentives.

- Current developments are aligning the incentives of three groups – payors, providers, and managed care organizations – into tight cooperative entities, aimed at reducing costs. Patients are excluded from such schemes.

- Some major ethical problems are partly the product of an economic structure that brings the economic incentives of physicians into harmony with those of the MCO, while leaving patients under a completely different set of incentives and, thereby, expectations.

- Whereas providers are rewarded for delivering a conservative level of care, patients' economic insulation encourages them to continue an Artesian mentality, often believing that health care is free and that they have an unlimited right to the best medical care, spare no expense.

- There are two levels on which to resolve the problems that arise from this situation – on the policy level, by including patients in resource decisions, and on the clinical level, by bringing them into the economic incentives that guide physicians, and MCOs.

- On the policy level, two things should be done: 1) patients should be thoroughly informed about the MCO's resource policies, such as incentive systems and other utilization controls; 2) policies governing what levels of care an MCO covers should be influenced, if not determined, by patients' participation in policy-making mechanisms.

- On the clinical level, patients need to be more immediately connected with the financial consequences of their care. Patients must join payors and providers in systems that reward the prudent use of resources.

- If patients had reason and reward for considering costs more carefully, there would be less need for outsiders to decide which care is worth its cost, and thereby less need for intrusive UR, and less gaming of the system.

A SUGGESTED PROCESS FOR REFLECTING ON THIS ARTICLE:

(see pages 234-254 for other processes that might better fit your specific goals and objectives).

Issue	What I like	What I don't like	How we could implement
Whereas providers are rewarded for delivering a conservative level of care, patients' economic insulation encourages them to continue an Artesian mentality, often believing that health care is free and that they have an unlimited right to the best medical care, spare no expense.			
There are two levels on which to resolve the problems that arise from this situation – on the policy level, by including patients in resource decisions, and on the clinical level, by bringing them into the economic incentives that guide physicians and MCOs.			
On the policy level, two things should be done: 1) patients should be thoroughly informed about the MCO's resource policies, such as incentive systems and other utilization controls; 2) policies governing what levels of care an MCO covers should be influenced, if not determined, by patients' participation in policy-making mechanisms.			
On the clinical level, patients need to be more immediately connected with the financial consequences of their care. Patients must join payors and providers in systems that reward the prudent use of resources.			
If patients had reason and reward for considering costs more carefully, there would be less need for outsiders to decide which care is worth its cost, and thereby less need for intrusive UR, and less gaming of the system.			

IN LIGHT OF OUR DISCUSSION:

*   as (executive committee, ethics committee, etc.), what are some next steps that we should take?

*   as (hospital, home health agency, etc.), what are some next steps that we should take?

*   what systems and structures call for special attention in order to improve the situation?

ENDNOTES

1. Hillman AL. Financial incentives for physician in HMOs: Is there a conflict of interest? *N. Eng. J. Med.* 1987; 317: 1743-1748; Levinson DF. Toward full disclosure of referral restrictions and financial incentives by prepaid health plans. *N. Eng. J. Med.* 1987; 317: 1729-1731; Berenson RA. In a doctor's wallet. *New Republic* 1987; 196: 11-13; Scovern H. A physician's experiences in a for-profit staff-model HMO. *N. Eng. J. Med.* 1988; 319:787-790; Povar G, Moreno J. Hippocrates and the health maintenance

organization: A discussion of ethical issues. *Ann Intern Med* 1988; 109:419-424; Morreim EH. Fiscal scarcity and the inevitability of bedside budget balancing. *Arch Intern Med* 1989; 149 (5):1012-1015; Morreim EH. Gaming the system: Dodging the rules, ruling the dodgers. *Arch Intern Med* 1991; 151 (3):443-447; Morreim EH. Cost containment: Challenging fidelity and justice. *Hastings C Rep* 1988; 18(6): 20-25.

2. Morreim EH. *Balancing act: The new medical ethics of medicine's new economics.* Dordrecht: Kluwer Academic Publishers, 1991; Butler SM, Haislmaier EF, eds. *Critical issues: A national health system for America.* Washington: The Heritage Foundation, 1989; Starr P. *The Social Transformation of American Medicine.* Basic Books, New York, 1982.

3. Morreim EH. "Redefining quality by reassigning responsibility"; *Am J Law Med* 1994; 20(1-2):79-104.

4. Morreim EH. Rationing and the law. In: *Rationing America's Medical Care: The Oregon Plan and Beyond.* Strosberg MA, Wiener JM, Baker R, and Fein IA, eds. Washington, D.C.: Brookings Institution, 1992, 159-184; Morreim EH. Stratified scarcity: Redefining the standard of care. *Law, Med and Health Care* 1989; 17(4):356-367; Morreim EH. Cost containment and the standard of medical care. *Calif L Rev* 1987;75 (5):1719-63.

5. Morreim EH. Balancing act, pp. 9-21.

6. Health Maintenance Organization Act of 1973 (42 U.S.C. §300e).

7. Morreim, Balancing Act, p. 33.

8. Blum JD. Economic credentialing: A new twist in hospital appraisal processes. *J Legal Med* 1991; 12:427-475; Bjornstad B, Mohlenbrock B. Economic credentialing in the era of integrated health care. In: *Integrated Health Care Delivery Systems,* Fine A, ed. New York: Thompson Publishing Group, Inc., 1993; 39-56; *Hassan v. Independent Practice Associates,* P.C., 698 F.Supp. 679 (E.D.Mich. 1988).

9. Sederer LI. Managed mental health care and professional compensation. *Behavioral Sciences and the Law* 1994; 12:367-78, at 367 (emphasis added).
Other commentators use similar language. "Aligning incentives across the organization is another key to success." Rogers MC, Snyderman R, Rogers EL. Cultural and organizational implications of academic managed-care networks. *N. Eng. J. Med.* 1994;331: 1374-77, at 1376; See also: Terry K. Is this the best way to divide HMO income? *MedEcon* 1994; 71(19):26B-26F, at 26D; Hall R.C. Social and legal implications of managed care in psychiatry. *Psychosomatics* 1994;34:150-158, at 150.

10. Sulmasy DP. Managed care and managed death. *Arch Intern Med* 1995; 155:133-136.

11. Morreim EH. Of rescue and responsibility: learning to live with limits. *J Med and Philos* 1994; 19:455-470; Morreim EH. Redefining quality by redefining responsibility; *Am J Law and Med* 1994; 20 (1-2): 79-104.

12. C. Havighurst. Prospective self-denial: can consumers contract today to accept health care rationing tomorrow? 140 *U Penn L Rev,* 1755, 1785 (1992); U. Reinhardt, American values: are they blocking health-system reform? 69 (21) *Med Econ,* 126, 141 (1992); U. Reinhardt, You pay when business bankrolls health care, *WSJ,* December 2, 1992, at A-14; J. Weaver, The best care other people's money can buy, *WSJ,* November 19, 1992, at A-14.

13. Azavedo D. Why can't other HMOs work as well as this one? *Med Econ* 1994; 71 (7):102-110.

14. Blendon RJ, Brodie M, Benson J. What should be done now that national health system reform is dead? *JAMA* 1995;273:243-44, at 243.

15. Patients also use such suits against MCOs and insurers to gain access to costly care they feel they deserve, even where it may not be covered by their policy. See Peters WP, Rogers MC. Variation in approval by insurance companies of coverage for autologous bone marrow transplantation for breast cancer. *N. Eng. J. Med.* 31994;330:473-477.

16. Miller RH, Luft HS. Managed care plan performance since 1980. *JAMA* 1994;271:1512-1519.

17. Morreim EH. Gaming the system: Dodging the rules, ruling the dodgers. *Arch Intern Med* 1991; 151 (3):443-447.

18. McCormick B. What price patient advocacy? *AMN,* 3/28/94,1,13.

19. The author goes on to observe that "[t]his was a bold demand for a company that a 1988 federal jury had found to have fixed prices, violated securities laws, and engaged in racketeering and which had drawn fire from its doctors for reducing authorized laboratory services and instituting a 'preferred drug' list." Wooley SC. Managed care and mental health: the silencing of a profession. *Internat J Eating Disorders* 1993; 14:387-401, at 394. See also: Orient J. *Your Doctor Is Not In: Healthy Skepticism about National Health Care*. New York: Crown Publishers Inc. 1994, at 159: "The details of that contract are generally kept secret from the patients, and for good reason. The contract might forbid the doctor to make derogatory comments about the plan. It will set forth the financial incentives that the gatekeeper has for denying or restricting care. It will delineate the barriers that the gatekeeper will have to overcome (phone calls, forms, committee meetings, etc.) in order to obtain approval for any unusual procedures he wants his patient to have."

20. Consumer-First Health Care (editorial). *WSJ*, 7/21/94; A-12.

21. Glover GJ, Kuhlik BN. Potential liability associated with restrictive drug policies. *Seton Hall Legis J* 1990;14:103-13.

22. *Moore v. Regents of the University of California*, 793 P.2d479 (Cal. 1990) (cert. denied 112 S. Ct. 2967(1992)); Morreim EH. Economic disclosure and economic advocacy: New duties in the medical standard of care. *J Legal Med* 1991;12(3):275-329.

23. Morreim, EH. Balancing act.

24. Figa SF, Tag HM. Redefining full and fair disclosure of HMO benefits and limitations. *Seton Hall Legis J* 1990;14:151-57; Chittenden WA. Malpractice liability and managed health care: History and prognosis. *Tort and Insurance Law J* 1991;26:451-496; Hirshfeld EB. Should third party payors of health care services disclose cost control mechanisms to potential beneficiaries? *Seton Hall Legis J* 1990; 14:115-150. The AMA now recommends requiring such disclosures. (Promises, promises: a proposed law would ensure managed care lives up to its sales pitch. AMN, 5/16/94, p. 19) A few states have proposed requiring such disclosures, but no such laws have passed as yet. See Jones M. Institutional liability for medical malpractice. In: Hall HA, ed. Health Care Corporate Law: Financing and Liability. Boston: Little, Brown, and Company, 1993. (chapter 8), at p. 8-65.

25. Chittenden WA. Malpractice liability and managed health care: History and prognosis. *Tort and Insurance Law J* 1991;26:451-496, at 475; Stern JB. Bad faith suits: are they applicable to health maintenance organizations? *W Virginia L Rev* 1983; 85:911-928; Povar G, Moreno J. Hippocrates and the health maintenance organization: A discussion of ethical issues. *Ann Intern Med* 1988; 109: 419-424. HMOs may even be seen as fiduciaries with respect to the physicians or other providers they enlist. See *Sanus/New York v. Dube-Seybold-Sutherland*, 837 S.W.2d 191 (Tex.App.-Houston [1st Dist.] 1992)

26. *Egan v Mutual of Omaha Ins Co.* 598 P.2d 452 (1979); *Davis v. Blue Cross of Northern California*, 600 P.2d 1060.

27. Tiano LV. The legal implications of HMO cost containment measures. *Seton Hall Legis J* 1990; 14:79-102; Chittenden WA. Malpractice liability and managed health care: History and prognosis. *Tort and Insurance Law J* 1991; 26: 451-496. Note that such suits are limited by ERISA law: if a health plan is obtained as an employment benefit, most such common-law causes of action are preempted in favor of much more limited Federal remedies.

28. Tiano LV. The legal implications of HMO cost containment measures. *Seton Hall Legis J* 1990;14:79-102; Chittenden WA. Malpractice liability and managed health care: History and prognosis. *Tort and Insurance Law J* 1991; 26:451-496. Meyer M and Murr A, Not my Health Care, *Newsweek,* 1/19/94, at 36-38; Pollock EJ. Jury tells HMO to pay damages in dispute over refused coverage. *WSJ* 12/28/93, B-4.

29. Younger PA, Conner C, Cartwright KK. *Managed Care Law Manual*. Gaithersburg: Aspen Publishers, Inc., 1994.

30. Azavedo D. Why can't other HMOs work as well as this one? *Med Econ* 1994;71(7): 102-110.

31. Azavedo D. Why can't other HMOs work as well as this one? *Med Econ* 1994;71(7): 102-110.

32. Gramm P. Why we need medical savings accounts. *N. Eng. J. Med.* 1994;330:1752-53.

33. Morreim EH. Of rescue and responsibility. *J Med and Philos* 1994;19:455-470; Morreim EH. Redefining quality by reassigning responsibility. *Am J Law and Med* 1994;20(1-2): 79-104.

34. Morreim, Of Rescue and responsibility. *Ibid.*

35. Rice B. Educate your pts without taking more time. *Med Econ* 1992 69(19):92-105; Barber BR. Participatory democracy in health care: the role of the responsible citizen. *Trends in Health Care, Law & Ethics* 1992; 7(3-4): 9-13; Shapiro RS, Simpson DE, Lawrence SL, Talsky AM, Sobocinski KA, Schiedermayer DL. A survey of sued and nonsued physicians and suing patients. *Arch Intern Med* 1989; 149:2190-2196; Redelmeier DA, Rozin P, Kahnerman D. Understanding patients' decisions: cognitive and emotional perspectives. *JAMA* 1993;270:72-76.

CHAPTER 12

ETHICAL CHARACTER OF HMO – KEY CHARACTERISTICS

John W. Glaser

From the various articles contained in this book, a number of issues are discussed that define the ethical quality of an MCO.

An ethically strong MCO should have explicit consensus about, commitment to, and effective systems and structures to realize values such as the following:

- Personal, long-term relationship between primary care provider and patients;

- Commitment to caring for the same population over time;

- Commitment to preventive care;

- Commitment to health promotion;

- Development of a consensus about the nature, purpose and key mechanisms of managed care among all key publics;

- Clear statements of rights and responsibilities for members, providers and the plan;

- The assurance that organizations with which the MCO has contracts have policies, procedures and practices that harmonize with their own;

- Recognition of cost containment as an essential of quality care;

- Systems to measure health outcomes;

- Strong physician involvement in guideline development;

- Culture of collaborative relationships and trust among primary care providers;

- Culture of collaborative relationships and trust between primary care providers and specialists;

- Profits maximally invested in health improvements of population;

- Financial incentives that include all concerned publics, including patients;

- Helps for employers to understand dimensions of managed care beyond price;

- Helps for employers to aid their employees in understanding managed care;
- Consensus on importance of population-based approach to health;
- Appropriate balance of mechanisms for cost-containment;
- Basis for financial incentives as outcomes-based rather than referals/utilization of services;
- Financial incentives spread over large groups;
- Financial incentives spread over longer, rather than shorter, time frames;
- Limits for ratio of at-risk to risk-free income;
- Clarification of the importance and role of tension between individual good and population good for all key publics;
- Commitment to continuous quality improvement;
- Systems to empower patients at key points: e.g., governance, guidelines, allocation and appeals;
- Systems to make shared responsibility of all key publics for population health visible and effective;
- Marketing that does not hide essential elements of managed care;
- Appropriate ratio of management costs to provision of care;
- Strong presence of physicians at key points: e.g., governance, guidelines development, allocation decisions, appeals;
- Preventive mechanisms for dealing with value/ethical concerns of staff/patients;
- Commitment of resources needed for communication and building of community;
- Systems and structures for continuous learning;
- Articulation of vision/values/philosophy;
- Systems and structures for implementation of vision/values/philosophy.

A SUGGESTED PROCESS FOR REFLECTING ON THIS ARTICLE:

(See pages 234-254 for other processes that might better fit your goals and objectives.)

Select your top ten from the above characteristics and put them in the order of importance – 1=most important 10=least important			
Issue	I personally agree	Verbal commitment by our organization	Actual Performance by our organization

IN LIGHT OF OUR DISCUSSION

- as (executive committee, ethics committee, etc.), what are some next steps that we should take?

- as (hospital, home health agency, etc.), what are some next steps that we should take?

- what systems and structures call for special attention in order to improve the situation?

PART 3

READINGS IN INDIVIDUAL
ETHICS OF MANAGED CARE

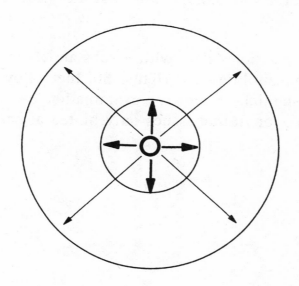

The articles in this section help us think about select questions of how individuals should understand and manage care. What are my duties and responsibilities concerning my own health? What do I owe other individuals, institutions and society concerning my own health? What do I owe other individuals, institutions and society concerning health care? How do these rights and responsibilities differ if I am a patient, nurse, physician, administrator, actuary, or marketer?

The following articles deal with a substantial but limited set of such responsibilities and rights. So, the following articles provide substantial content for examination but also can be a springboard for further issues only hinted at here.

CHAPTER 13

FACING THE ETHICAL CHALLENGES OF MANAGED CARE

Leonard M. Fleck, PhD, and Harriet Squier, MD, MA

WHILE YOU CAN DO A LOT TO PREVENT ETHICAL PROBLEMS, THE ETHICAL challenge at the heart of managed care won't go away.

While evidence shows increasingly that managed care systems can provide high-quality, cost-effective care with excellent outcomes, many physicians wonder if these systems have ethical costs or ethical risks that are too high. When considering whether to participate in a managed care organization (MCO), you need to examine the personal, professional and social ethical values that are important to you in your current practice, and reflect on how these might be challenged in a managed care environment. Since the ethical basis of one MCO may be more solid than that of another, you may be able to avoid putting yourself in an ethically intolerable position if you study the issues – and the organization – before you join.

SOURCES OF MORAL CONFLICT IN MANAGED CARE

Although all medical settings can generate ethical conflicts between patient interests and physician interests, managed care systems may make these conflicts more overt, more frequent and more complex, partly because third-party institutional interests suffuse virtually every aspect of the doctor-patient relationship. An MCO will encourage physicians to prescribe according to formulary guidelines, to refer to physicians on a provider panel, to shorten or avoid hospital stays, and generally to comply with guidelines and benefit limits for mental health services, specialty care and ancillary services. In staff-model MCOs, physicians may also be expected to see a minimum number of patients.[1]

Many MCOs are able to document that when physicians adhere to practice guidelines and provide cost-effective care, health outcomes are excellent and do not decline, despite patients' more limited access to specialty care, hospital care and expensive tests and treatments.[2] Nevertheless, many family physicians are uncomfortable about the restrictions MCOs tend to place on patient care. Physicians see themselves as loyal and uncompromised advocates of each patient's best interests. They see this responsibility as an ethical imperative at the core of medicine. But guidelines, by their nature, are about averages and aggregates of patients. It is that insensitivity to the unique needs and interests of individual patients that provokes the moral discomfort.

More precisely, ethical conflicts in managed care may concern restrictions on patient autonomy, a central value in contemporary medical ethics – restrictions that protect the economic interests of the physician or the MCO. They may also concern restrictions on physician autonomy that might compromise the welfare of patients and the moral integrity of physicians to protect the interests of the MCO.

ORGANIZATIONAL INTERESTS CAN BE PATIENT INTERESTS

Strictly speaking, an *ethical* conflict requires two ethical values to be in conflict. If an organizational self-interest threatens patient rights or physicians' moral integrity, then the ethical thing to do is obvious. Often enough, however, organizational interests in efficiency and cost-containment have more than an economic quality. When an organization's policy accurately reflects its members' choices, organizational interests possess a moral quality as well.

As countless opinion polls have shown, the majority of us want high-quality health care, and we want the costs contained at reasonable levels. In the ideal case, we turn to MCOs for health care, hoping to strike a balance between these dual interests. In becoming plan members, we agree with the other members on a set of rules and practices that will define legitimate access to a common pool of resources. In effect, these rules define the fair, or *just*, restricted claim that any one of us has to those resources. As long as we join a plan in full understanding of the choice we are making, our acceptance of the MCO's terms lends a fundamental moral quality to what would otherwise appear to be merely economic interests of the organization.

It's true, of course, that not every member of a managed care plan has freely joined the MCO – for instance, some individuals are in a plan because their employers chose that plan. While this is regrettable, it does not give any special moral rights to these individuals, such as exemptions from restrictions other plan members must follow. It does, however, create stronger moral obligations for physicians in the plan to educate patients early on about plan restrictions. Patients who find the restrictions unacceptable will at least have an adequate opportunity to explore other supplementary health care options. But plan members must acknowledge that while their physician has a responsibility to care for them, that responsibility is tempered by the responsibility to use the limited resources of the MCO prudently.

Physicians, in their role as expert judges of medical need in managed care plans, must be fair and impartial implementors of the rules of what we might call *prudent caring* for their patients, who (we assume) agreed to them freely. A physician in an MCO cannot be an *unrestricted advocate* of each patient's best interests. That is, a physician's advocacy can never ignore the needs of the rest of the MCO's members. Rather, the physician must be a *just* and *caring* advocate of each patient's interest – one who takes the patient's interests to heart but allows his or her advocacy of those interests to be limited by a sense of justice to the other patients in the plan. Striking a reasonable balance between justice and caring is the basic and inescapable ethical challenge posed by managed care, even by the best-run and fairest of managed care plans. A related challenge is to avoid other ethical problems – ones that are not inescapable – and that's where preventive ethics comes in.

THE PROMISE OF PREVENTIVE ETHICS

Medicine is often divided into preventive, acute and chronic modes. Medical ethics is appropriately thought of in the same terms. "Acute ethics" is probably the most common of the medical ethics modes. But recently, we have learned a lot about the importance of preventive ethics.

Decisions about withdrawing life-sustaining care from an incompetent patient are clearly among the most difficult and agonizing moral decisions physicians face today. Not knowing whether the patient would approve of your choice is morally perilous. But watching the patient endure the excruciating and dehumanizing terminal suffering that your medical decisions may prolong is morally intolerable. In principle, these situations can be avoided through timely communication about advance directives between patients and their primary care physicians. This is preventive ethics.

In the realm of managed care, there are many opportunities for the judicious use of preventive ethics. The first one arises when you consider becoming a provider in a particular MCO. Here are some strategic questions that will help you make a moral assessment of the plan and your role in it:

Have I reviewed the advertising of this MCO and considered whether it might mislead potential plan members in a way that is likely to generate moral problems for me in practice?

Several years ago, a full-page advertisement in *The Detroit Free Press* depicted a young mother holding a year-old baby. The headline read: "Medical care for this child cost $93,178, and Michigan HMO paid every penny." No one contemplating joining this HMO would conclude from such an advertisement that there were any limits on their access to medical care in this plan.

Have I carefully reviewed the budget of the MCO, with an especially critical eye for administrative and advertising expenses (and its profit margins, if it is a for-profit MCO)?

Physicians can, in good conscience, abide by rationing protocols that compromise patient welfare when they know that patients have agreed to those protocols, *and that the savings achieved will be used to meet higher priority, just claims to health services made by other plan members.* However, if 30% of the plan's dollars are used for something other than health care services, then physicians must wonder if they are really being loyal patient advocates when they abide by guidelines that deny their patients marginally beneficial care. Denying an elderly patient an extra day in the hospital after a serious heart attack so the MCO can purchase another 15-second TV spot is hardly a worthy activity of a loyal patient advocate.

Would my moral and professional integrity be seriously compromised by acting in accord with this MCO's cost-control mechanisms?

In particular, have I carefully examined the economic incentives used by the MCO that would directly affect my clinical practice, and have I asked myself if those incentives could reshape my clinical judgment in ways that inappropriately compromise good patient care? Might the incentives for limiting referrals to other specialists be such that I would manage some cases longer than I should?

Again, an important reminder: excessive testing, unnecessary hospital days and unnecessary specialty referrals can have unacceptable medical, economic and moral costs. Economic incentives for a conservative approach to therapy, closely tied to solid outcomes, should be seen as morally meritorious. In practice, however, incentive systems of various MCOs may be a complex mix of appropriate and dubiously appropriate incentives. There are no simple rules for sorting out these incentives. What you can do, however, is have in mind 10 or so situations that represent difficult cases from your practice, then think through how management of these cases might be affected by the incentive system of a given MCO, and judge whether these adjustments would prove morally troubling.

To what extent are plan physicians directly and effectively in charge of developing, critically assessing and authorizing cost-control mechanisms, such as clinical protocols or incentive systems, that directly affect the practice of medicine?

To the extent that such decisions are primarily a product of bottom-line business thinking by nonclinicians, the likelihood of daily challenges to the moral and professional integrity of the plan's physicians increases. The practical question you need to ask is whether you are willing to invest time and effort on review committees that assess cost-control mechanisms from the point of view of cost-conscious but just and caring physicians.

To what extent does the organizational culture of the MCO strongly support the core elements of a physician ethic of loyalty to patient interests?

Or to what extent is the "organization" a mere collection of physicians and managers brought together to protect their own economic interests? An increasing number of physicians find themselves coerced by economic circumstances into affiliating with an MCO.[3] This situation is less than ideal for conscientiously assessing an MCO from the viewpoint of how just and caring physicians ought to practice medicine.

To what extent are patients educated, before joining the plan, that for the sake of cost-control they are buying an approach to health services delivery that includes limits and trade-offs?

In particular, do representatives of the MCO explain to health care purchasers (and do they help employers explain to their employees) the plan's system of incentives and rules for controlling costs and limiting access to care? Further, are physicians in the plan encouraged to reveal to patients needing care, then and there, the specific constraints that will affect their access to care? Respect for patient autonomy requires such revelations, according to the AMA Council on Ethical and Judicial Affairs.[4] Denials of care are especially easy to conceal from patients because patients are unfamiliar with the practice of medicine. Physicians have a fiduciary relation to patients that requires that such denials and limitations be explained so patients can make an informed choice about how to respond. (See "Identifying ethical managed care organizations" for a summary of these questions.)

Finally, there are opportunities for a preventive ethics strategy to be put to work after you have joined the MCO, typically in the form of very simple and ordinary efforts at patient education. If you are going to adopt a more conservative, "watchful waiting" attitude toward a patient's medical problem, perhaps because this is part of a practice guideline in your MCO, then you should explain to the patient that the approach is *more likely* to protect both their medical and economic interests, with deliberate emphasis on *more likely* so that patients can begin to appreciate the ineradicable uncertainty that is part of medicine.

BALANCING COMPETING MORAL VALUES

While your best efforts at preventive ethics can protect you from unnecessary ethical problems, they can't insulate you from the central ethical challenge of managed care. The following case illustrates the inescapable conflict in being both just and caring in any managed care plan:

> You see a new patient in your office, a 27-year-old computer programmer who is manic-depressive. He has a number of self-destructive behaviors, an abusive family, some unresolved childhood issues and a limited income. You know he would benefit from frequent visits with a psychiatrist for both behavioral and medication management, but the mental health benefits of his HMO are very limited. He is reluctant to establish a relationship with any mental health professional because he becomes depressed easily and became suicidal after a previous therapist left town. He requests that you manage all his psychiatric care, even though your training in this area is somewhat limited.

Several courses of action are open to you, all more or less acceptable, but none really satisfying from an ethical perspective:

1. You could advise the patient to seek the expert psychiatric care he needs and pay the extra costs himself, despite the financial hardship and the patient's aversion to psychiatric help.

2. You could initiate whatever appeals are necessary to convince the HMO to cover the costs of long-term, out-of network psychiatric care for the patient, despite your awareness that the appeal process will take a good deal of your time and that the HMO denies a large percentage of such appeals.

3. You could manage the patient's psychiatric care yourself, despite your awareness that counseling is not your strong suit and your belief that the patient would benefit more from seeing a psychiatrist.

4. You could refer the patient for whatever mental health services the HMO will pay for, despite knowing that those services are very limited, and again despite the patient's wish to have you manage his care.

Option I is morally attractive because you would be recommending what is medically best for the patient, while not diverting HMO resources from other members with just claims on them. The downside is that this is not what the patient wants. He does not see this option as being in his best interest, when that best interest includes accepting financial hardship as well as the feelings of psychological insecurity. You could try to persuade him to reconsider what is in his long-term best interest, but this could still leave you in a bind. As you watch his financial resources be consumed in psychiatric care, might you not be asking yourself whether your recommendation has deprived him of HMO benefits that are justly his? (What, after all, does the HMO owe him? It provides the appeal process specifically to give deserving patients access to extraordinary services. Are you ethically justified in denying him his opportunity to appeal?)

Option 2 is more attractive at least because it would allow you to be a strong patient advocate by vigorously working to get your patient the care you believe is in his best interests, while responding to some of his concerns. On the downside, it would require several hours of your time to write the letters and make the phone call us the appeal process requires. And you know from experience that there is no more than, say, a 30% chance of a successful appeal.

Are you morally obligated to invest this much of your personal and professional time on behalf of one patient, given that you have many other patients with legitimate claims to your time? While no patient has a moral right to make unlimited demands on a physician's time, physicians have a moral obligation to make special efforts for patients with special needs. Ultimately, this will be a matter of reasonable moral judgment. Your time would be less of a factor if the appeal were more likely to succeed. But while you might be able to ensure success by choosing words that would shade the diagnosis to convey a more serious problem than you think the patient has, that is dishonest, and it corrupts the rules plan members agreed to regarding just access to benefits.

Option 3 now looks somewhat attractive. If one of the cardinal moral principles in medical ethics is respect for patient autonomy, then Option 3 has much to recommend it. The patient wants you to manage his psychological problems as well as his other medical problems, and this option respects the just limits plan members agreed to. The moral downside is that you are acutely conscious of the fact that you are not a psychiatrist. You have enough counseling skills that you won't likely make the patient feel worse, but you doubt your ability to make him better. If you are supposed to be a loyal and uncompromised advocate of the best interests of your patient, is this course morally acceptable? There is also the issue of your time and compensation. These are not 15-minute office visits. These are likely to be half-hour and hour-long sessions, for which you receive neither additional compensation nor release from patient-volume expectations. To what extent is it morally permissible for you to allow these considerations of self-interest to compromise your role as a patient advocate?

Option 4 also has morally attractive features. It rests on the reasonable premise that members of the MCO agreed to, presumably of their own free will: that no one in this MCO has an unlimited moral right to its resources, including the time of the physicians who serve the plan. Everyone's just claims to common resources are justly limited by the just claims of everyone else in the plan. The patient can receive competent mental health care that is suitable to his needs, but it will not be the best care and perhaps not the most appropriate care. Although we might all prefer to have access to superior quality medicine, this is clearly an unreasonable expectation that has no moral force. Still, Option 4 seems less than satisfactory, morally speaking, partly because it is less than respectful of this patient's autonomous choices, and partly because it makes you feel like a half-hearted, less-than-loyal patient advocate. It still begs the question of what the patient's just claims are. He clearly has a special need, but does that need justify the special expenditure of HMO resources?

Do you find the situation frustrating? You're not alone. All four options seem, morally speaking, to be less than satisfactory, or at best, merely satisfactory. Surely a just and caring physician should be able to do better than to end up in such a moral swamp. If managed care consistently yielded moral mediocrity, that in itself would be a powerful argument against managed care. But the solution needn't be to abolish managed care. On the contrary, we believe that, with the help of virtuous managed care organizations, physicians can rise above this sort of moral mediocrity. To do so, however, requires ingenuity, dedication and constant moral diligence by physicians – and an abiding commitment by MCOs to map out ethical pathways that lead out of the swamp. Make no mistake: doctors will have great difficulty being just and caring patient advocates in organizations that are assiduously amoral.

THE NEED FOR VIRTUOUS ORGANIZATIONS

Ethical problems are often thought of as value conflicts that individuals must wrestle with in the privacy of their own conscience. We would argue that this is not true of medical ethics in general, and certainly not of the ethical issues that characterize managed care. These issues need to be talked through and thought out in public forums that are part of the managed care organization *and that have the capacity to shape the policies and practices of that organization*. It is through this process that virtuous organizations are created and sustained. The questions raised by the case we've just reviewed are not the kind to be answered by one person. The ethical justification for managed care is the fair distribution of limited resources, and fairness is impossible unless all players agree on what's fair. Before the questions can be answered satisfactorily, we need a more elaborate and generally accepted ethical infrastructure for managed care than we now have.

What would you do?

Your patient is a 52-year-old man with headaches that are suspicious enough that a CT scan is warranted. As you explain the procedure, you mention that a dye will be injected into him to give a better image. He recalls a neighbor of his "who nearly died when they put that cheap dye in him. They should have used the more expensive stuff." He wants assurances from you that he will get that safer, more expensive dye. You know that the policy of your MCO is to use high-osmolality contrast agents, unless medical history dictates otherwise. You also know that your patient was forced into retirement by heart disease and has a very limited income. He could not afford the added cost of a low osmolality contrast agent. Morally speaking, what should you say or do as a just and caring patient advocate?

Many hospitals today have institutional ethics committees which, when functioning properly, can serve as the conscience of the organization. MCOs that would be virtuous need comparable entities. The ethics committee of an MCO should, first of all, be a forum for the reflective critical discussion and resolution of moral conflicts that emerge within the organization, such as that of our computer programmer – a forum that is easily accessible to patients, providers and managers. Second, the committee should provide the organizational matrix for the development of the policies and practices that will define and protect the character of the organization as a whole.

An MCO ethics committee must have explicit responsibility for critically evaluating all the organization's policies and practices associated with cost-containment from a moral point of view (the perspective of what a just and caring, trustworthy and honest organization ought to be). Among other things, the committee should see to it that incentive systems for shaping physician behavior are carefully reviewed for their effects on physician integrity and patient welfare, that rationing protocols are explicit and well-known to patients, both at the time of enrollment and when care is needed, that rationing protocols are fairly implemented, that administrative expenses are strictly controlled so that maximal dollars flow to patient care, that advertising is not misleading, and so on.

Finally, a managed care ethics committee has a serious educational responsibility. Ethical guidelines, policies and practices are nothing more than window dressing if providers and managers do not understand them and are therefore not motivated to carry them out. This is no small challenge. Academic ethicists are familiar with the fundamental moral challenge, "Why be moral?" It is usually viewed as an interesting theoretical question. In the intensely competitive world of managed care, the question demands a practical, feasible answer.

Physicians as members of a profession must grapple with this question and come up with a compelling response. They must figure out how a virtuous managed care organization can survive in a competitive health care system, and must maintain individual ethical commitments with a core defined by the medical profession as a whole. Failure to do so will undermine the future capacity of physicians in managed care to be either just or caring patient advocates.

KEY IDEAS IN THIS ARTICLE:

- The majority of us want high-quality health care, and we want the costs contained at reasonable levels.

- We turn to MCOs hoping to strike a balance between these dual interests. In becoming members, we agree with the other members on a set of rules and practices that will define legitimate access to a common pool of resources.

- A physician in an MCO cannot be an *unrestricted* advocate of each patient's best interest, but must also attend to the needs of the rest of the MCO's members.

- Some strategic questions to help make an ethical assessment of the plan and an individuals role in it:

  - Have I reviewed the advertising of this MCO and considered whether it might mislead potential plan members in a way that is likely to generate moral problems for me in practice?

  - Have I carefully reviewed the budget of the MCO, with an especially critical eye for administrative and advertising expenses (and its profit margins, if it is a for-profit MCO)?

  - Would my moral and professional integrity be seriously compromised by acting in accord with this MCO's cost-control mechanisms?

  - To what extent are the plan physicians directly and effectively in charge of developing, critically assessing and authorizing cost-control mechanisms, such as clinical protocols or incentive systems, that directly affect the practice of medicine?

  - To what extent does the organizational culture of the MCO strongly support the core elements of a physician's ethic of loyalty to patient interests?

  - To what extent are patients educated, before joining the plan, that for the sake of cost-control they are buying an approach to health services delivery that includes limits and trade-offs?

A SUGGESTED PROCESS FOR REFLECTING ON THIS ARTICLE:

(see pages 234-254 for other processes that might better fit your specific goals and objectives).

Issue:	Is clearly an ethical good 1-5 5=high	Degree of feasibility	Steps to make it more feasible
1. We turn to MCOs hoping to strike a balance between these dual interests. In becoming members, we agree with the other members on a set of rules and practices that will define legitimate access to a common pool of resources.			
2. A physician in an MCO cannot be an unrestricted advocate of each patient's best interest, but must also attend to the needs of the rest of the MCO's members.			

Issue:	Is clearly an ethical good 1-5 5=high	Degree of feasibility	Steps to make it more feasible
3. I have carefully reviewed the budget of the MCO, with an especially critical eye for administrative and advertising expenses (and its profit margins, if it is a for-profit MCO).			
4. Patients are educated, before joining the plan, that for the sake of cost-control they are buying an approach to health services delivery that includes limits and trade-offs.			
5. Physicians are directly and effectively in charge of developing, critically assessing and authorizing cost-control mechanisms, such as clinical protocols or incentive systems, that directly affect the practice of medicine.			

IN LIGHT OF OUR DISCUSSION:

- as (executive committee, ethics committee, etc.), what are some next steps that we should take?

- as (hospital, home health agency, etc.), what are some next steps that we should take?

- what systems and structures call for special attention in order to improve the situation?

ENDNOTES

1. Rodwin MA. Conflicts in managed care. *N Engl J Med* 1995;332:604-607.
2. Miller RH, Luft HS. Managed care plan performance since 1980. *JAMA* 1994;271:1512-1519.
3. Kassirer JP. Managed care and the morality of the marketplace. *N Eng J Med* 1995;333:50-52.
4. Council on Ethical and Judicial Affairs, AMA. Ethical issues in managed care. *JAMA* 1995;273:330-335.

CHAPTER 14

PHYSICIANS, COST CONTROL, AND ETHICS

Daniel P. Sulmasy, OFM, MD

Rising health care expenditures have led to numerous cost-control proposals. An examination of the ethical questions surrounding the role that physicians play in the control of health care costs suggests that unilateral rationing decisions by individual physicians at the bedside are morally unacceptable. Such decisions are arbitrary, ineffective in redistributing health care resources, and formally unjust. Restrictive gatekeeping (the creation of financial incentives for physicians to limit care given to individual patients) also seems unacceptable because of its morally significant effects. First, it disguises the role of those actually responsible for cost-control decisions; second, it routinely creates a "moral stress test" by forcing physicians to act in ways that are contrary to their own interests in order to serve the needs of patients; third, it undermines the trust between doctor and patient; and fourth, it rations by class of persons rather than class of technology. In contrast, a morally sound system would attempt to control costs by honestly informing patients and assigning responsibility justly, would encourage physicians to act in the interests of patients, would foster trust, and would recognize the great importance of equal treatment for all patients. Such a system would depend on input from an informed public and would apply equally to all members of society.

Annals of Internal Medicine, 1992;116:920-926

The doctor is, de facto, a gatekeeper. Access to the tests and treatments of contemporary, scientific American medicine is granted only through the powerful pen of the physician. The physician has traditionally been considered to have a moral obligation to use that power for the good of the patient, using only the tests and treatments needed to help that patient. Rising health care costs, however, have precipitated a line of reasoning which concludes that this de facto gatekeeping role should be expanded. Some have suggested that the physician should take social needs into account at the bedside, and make unilateral rationing decisions. Others believe that physicians should be restrictive gatekeepers, with institutionalized incentives for controlling costs. I argue that both bedside rationing and restrictive gatekeeping are morally illegitimate roles for the physician. In the course of this discussion, the terms cost-control, rationing, de facto gatekeeping, restrictive gatekeeping, fee for service, factitious gatekeeping, and salary are used extensively. Explicit definitions of these terms, as used here, are given in the Appendix.

THE PROBLEM

Health care now accounts for about 12% of the gross national product (GNP) of the United States[1] and is expected to climb to 16% by the year 2000.[2] Much of our health care bill is felt to be the result of the many technologically innovative, but expensive and perhaps only marginally effective diagnostic and therapeutic modalities available to patients in the U.S. The injudicious use of tests and treatments by American physicians is also responsible for these high costs. The demonstration of regional variations in the rates of utilization of health care resources is often cited as evidence of this problem.[3] Those who propose the implementation of stringent cost-control measures are generally motivated by the concern that society is currently spending too much money on health care, while many other projects, such as education, or the struggle against crime and drugs, remain woefully underfunded. They argue that attempts to merely "trim the fat" from health care expenditures have been inadequate, and that "strong medicine"[4] is necessary. They claim that such cost-control measures are preferable because they make explicit the situations that have implicitly controlled costs in this country for years: cost-control through the limitation of access to care by geographical and financial barriers.

Many think that the time for rationing health care is long overdue.[5,6] Others have argued that the conditions under which it will be necessary to ration health care have not yet been fully realized in the United States.[7,8] The intent of this paper is not to engage in such debate, nor to argue for any particular system of health care delivery. The aim is instead to suggest, from an ethical perspective, the role that physicians should play in any system that decides to explicitly control health care costs, and to critique some current proposals.

A MORAL SYSTEM OF COST CONTROL: PRINCIPLES

Both physicians and patients must acknowledge that no resource, including health care, is unlimited. In the face of rising expenditures, cost-control measures that do not include rationing, such as improved education, more effective peer review, and reduced administrative costs, should be considered first-line measures. Rationing becomes a morally acceptable option if the need is great enough, and if other methods have been exhausted.

This discussion assumes that a role-specific morality exists internal to the practice of medicine and operates under a model of beneficence in trust.[9] I contend that any cost-control system must acknowledge and support a relationship of trust between doctor and patient, and that the system should encourage cost-control through reform of the medical profession, rather than build upon physicians' vices. This argument carries the assumption that a moral sound cost-control system would preferably ration by classes of technology, and not by classes of persons. Decisions about what is to be rationed ought to be made matters of open public debate, and decision-makers should be identifiable and responsible to the public. Finally, physicians should responsibly provide this public debate with honest information about the actual burdens and benefits to be expected from emerging technologies. This essay evaluates several cost-control proposals as they relate to the previously mentioned principles.

WHY NO PHYSICIAN SHOULD MAKE UNILATERAL RATIONING DECISIONS

Physicians frequently argue that certain procedures should be withheld from particular patients because such interventions are felt to waste money that would be better spent elsewhere. Encouraging physicians to act on such thoughts might be one way to control costs, but this approach is morally problematic.

To see why this is so, imagine a physician, Doctor No, who realizes that many worthwhile programs in preventive medicine and a variety of important programs outside of medicine are woefully underfunded. Suppose that on this basis, Dr. No decides that he is justified in withholding certain diagnostic and therapeutic technologies from patients, expressly to conserve resources for preventive medicine and other services. Suppose that Dr. No assumes the care of Ms. Jones, a 25-year-old mentally retarded woman who, as a result of cerebral palsy, has been quadriplegic since birth. Imagine that Ms. Jones has been receiving parenteral nutrition for a year. She cannot be fed enternally because her intestines infarcted during an attempted jejunostomy tube placement, which was done after she had repeated bouts of aspiration pneumonia. Ms. Jones smiles and coos and interacts with her father, who has provided 25 years of dedicated care. Her father expects her care to continue. But after her third episode of central venous line sepsis within a year, Dr. No decides to provide no further therapy because the money can be better spent elsewhere. Why is this approach morally unacceptable?

First, it has not been established to everyone's satisfaction that the conditions necessitating health care rationing have been met. It is not impossible, for example, for society to increase tax revenues to simultaneously fund both health care and other projects. Further, everyone might not agree with Dr. No's choices of which treatments and tests to limit, and for whom they should be limited. Dr. No would need to justify to everyone else why he alone should make these decisions.

Second, it remains to be proven that the proposed action by Dr. No, even if generalized to include the practices of all physicians, would actually result in the redistribution of funds to the causes that Dr. No believes are more worthwhile. Effective redistribution would be extraordinarily improbable in a non-nationalized health care system.

Third, suppose Dr. No does make the decision, based on perceived societal needs, not to treat his patient, Ms. Jones. Suppose that Dr. No's colleague, Dr. Yes, never makes microallocational decisions based on perceived societal needs, and that Dr. Yes, therefore, gives antibiotics and a new central line to her mentally retarded 25-year-old patient, Mr. Smith, who has cerebral palsy and recurrent episodes of line sepsis. Under these circumstances, Ms. Jones has, de facto, been dealt an injustice under an Aristotelian[10] principle of formal justice (assuming that Ms. Jones and Mr. Smith are otherwise similar in relevant medical characteristics and that the proposed intervention is medically indicated and beneficial for both). The only way to avoid this injustice would be to use an explicit, societally accepted rule for allocation made at higher levels of social organization, so that all physicians would make it their goal to treat all similar patients equally under that rule.

This argument does not imply that all unequal treatment represents a formal injustice. When physicians honestly disagree in matters of clinical judgment, but agree on the principle of mobilizing resources for the good of each patient according to the patient's need, unequal treatment of similar patients may occur without injustice. In such cases, physicians intend to treat equals equally, but disagree in their judgments about differences in the conditions of patients who are later found to be, in fact, equivalent. Such physicians may be wrong, but as long as they are not culpably ignorant in their judgments about the patients, they are not acting unjustly. In our health care system, however, intentional decisions to limit interventions made unilaterally by individual practitioners for reasons of cost-control will necessarily be made with the expectation that other physicians will treat similar patients differently. Such unilateral decisions are, therefore, inherently inequitable and arbitrary, and should not be tolerated.

WHY PHYSICIANS SHOULD NOT BE RESTRICTIVE GATEKEEPERS

Although unilateral bedside rationing seems unacceptable, other cost-control measures might be preferable. For example, many good reasons seem to support the incorporation of restrictive gatekeeping into the health care system. It seems reasonable to make the de facto gatekeepers, the physicians, into restrictive gatekeepers by instituting financial incentives for physicians to control costs. The cause is noble, the means seem upright and straightforward, and the need to control costs seems acute. Yet, significant objections exist.

Disguising the Decision Maker

The first objection to such incentive plans is that restrictive gatekeeping makes it difficult for the public to understand who is responsible for rationing. By placing the locus of decision-making in the hands of physicians, policymakers unload the unpleasant task of deciding who should not receive various health care interventions. When physicians assume the role of the proximate decision-makers in limiting diagnosis and therapy on purely economic grounds, the role of the ultimate decision-makers (the policymakers) becomes ambiguous. Such ambiguity will exist regardless of whether these decision-makers are the board of a nonprofit hospital, a for-profit health maintenance organization (HMO), members of Congress, a state Medicaid administration, or an agency administrating a system of national health insurance. If patients are to be respected as persons, they should be informed of exactly who is limiting therapy. Policy architects might feel more comfortable when they do not need to face a crowd of protesting patients who have been cut off from a treatment program, but because the decision to control medical costs must be made societally, the decisions about where to cut should also be made societally. Rationing decisions, to be just, should follow a process of public debate in which widely promulgated proposals are discussed before enactment. Similarly, patients who join an HMO should know exactly which services will, and which will not, be covered.[11] An administrative decision to control costs by making physicians restrictive gatekeepers is, thus, in a subtle but significant fashion, a failure on the part of administrators to bear honestly their proper responsibility to inform the public.

Rationing by Classes of People

Some favor restrictive gatekeeping by physicians over categorical rationing because the former allows physicians to adjust the distribution of benefits to individual patients.[12] This approach overlooks a serious problem. As a general principle, when a disorder is common, and a new therapy or diagnostic tool is marginally superior but much more expensive than current modalities, it seems more equitable and just to ration by withholding this class of technology (call it X) from everyone, rather than to decide that technology X will be made available to some patients, but not to others. If one decides to allow only selected patients access to technology X, one must have a method for choosing among those who could benefit. One could decide, for example, to ration by mental status, so that those able to count by serial sevens would receive technology X, but that persons with Down syndrome would not. One might decide instead, for example, to ration by expected utility, and therefore to treat only nondiabetic patients who would, on average, live for 10 years with benefit from technology X, but not to treat diabetic patients, who would only survive for an average of five years. A third approach would be to adopt a restrictive gatekeeping system and leave it to each doctor to decide, by his own private and secret formula (ultimately based on his own income), who should receive technology X. All these methods seem unjust compared with the statement that "technology X is expensive, and only marginally better than Y. Let's not let anyone have technology X, so that we can spend the money on technology Z for everyone."

A Moral Stress Test for Physicians

A modest degree of altruism has traditionally been expected of all physicians as professionals.[13] But physicians are human. In a system of restrictive gatekeeping, physicians are forced continually into a series of moral stress tests, knowing that the consequences of doing good for patients will either entail financial penalties for themselves or limit the resources available to other patients. No one should be surprised if physicians readily succumb to excessive temptations to put their interests ahead of those of patients, because this is precisely the behavior expected in restrictive gatekeeping. The presumption of physician self-interest as the societally condoned means of cost-control undermines the traditional expectation of altruism. The allurement of physicians to control costs by acting in self-interest makes it more difficult for physicians to strive for the ideal that patient needs must come first.

The Disruption of Trust

A policy that makes physicians restrictive gatekeepers disrupts the trust central to the doctor-patient relationship. Even if physicians "pass" the moral stress test and little evidence accumulates that patients are grossly harmed by restrictive gatekeeping, the appearance of such a system will further erode the declining sense of trust between doctor and patient. The policy architects advocating restrictive gatekeeping will have transformed a relationship in which the physician has traditionally been regarded as a patient advocate into one in which the patient and physician assume adversarial roles in a struggle between proximate economic rivals. In a system of restrictive gatekeeping, an honest doctor might say to her dyspneic and frightened patient with a PO_2 of 56 mm Hg, "No, you can't have oxygen at home because I need the money to send my children to college." A less-honest physician might say "Oxygen won't help you." It would be less-disruptive to the doctor-patient relationship to abandon restrictive gatekeeping in favor of an explicit, public rule. Then, even if the system rationed by class of persons rather than by class of technology, at least the doctor could say, "I'm on your side. I'd like to help you, but I can't. No one with your level of blood oxygen is allowed to get oxygen at home. I know that oxygen would make you feel better, and please be assured that I would give it to you if I could, but it's against the rules. Perhaps we should both campaign to have the rules changed, for your sake and for the sake of others like you."

The patient, already made vulnerable by disease and the lack of medical expertise, is at increased risk for exploitation in a system of restricted gatekeeping. The patient must always be wary that the physician may be overstretching her competence to avoid making a costly referral or may withhold a treatment because of personal financial considerations. The disruption of trust, structurally part of restrictive gatekeeping, would be too high a price to pay for cost saving.

Salaries, Capitation, and Restrictive Gatekeeping

Financial incentives alone are not the problem. Similar questions also arise in other capitation arrangements, such as pre-paid individual practice-type HMOs,[14] and salary-type independent practice-type associations.[15] In these arrangements, physicians are prospectively allocated a fixed amount of money to expend on health care for the patients capitated to them, despite the fact that the physicians are, in essence, paid fixed salaries. Such capitation strategies constitute a form of gatekeeping, because the money spent to help one patient may limit the funds remaining to help others in the capitation group. In such systems, informed patients could justifiably worry that they were competing with every person in the waiting room, and they might be wary of the physician who could be forced to decide, without explicit, public criteria, who among the competing patients will receive needed medical care.

Systems that simply assign a group of patients to each physician under a fixed budget for the care of that group ask each physician to decide how big a slice of pie to cut for each patient. Because the size of the budget is fixed, treatment or diagnosis for one patient has the resources available for the next. If one patient assigned to the physician develops an anemia that is responsive to erythropoietin, the physician must decide not whether such expensive treatment would improve the patient's well-being, but whether such beneficial treatment would limit the funds available in the capitation pool for pneumococcal vaccination of his elderly patients. Informed elderly patients might resent the fact that their capitation group contained large numbers of patients at high-risk for renal failure and at risk for requiring expensive treatments, like dialysis and erythropoietin. Bias by the physician or among patients thus becomes an ever-present and insidious threat.

Further, the size of the risk pool is important. The risk may be assumed by the physician (in systems in which physician income is derived directly from capitated funds), or it may be assumed only by the patients whose fees are capitated to the pool of funds used for their care. In either case, smaller-risk pools make physicians more cost-conscious. Although smaller-risk pools can save more money, peculiar injustices can result. Some capitation schemes break the health care system down into little, isolated resource ponds. For example, every patient in a prepaid plan might be assigned to one primary care practitioner, with a fixed amount of money per patient assigned to that physician to use in caring for that group of patients. Supposing that the total health care system could accommodate two bone marrow transplant patients, both might be assigned to the same primary care capitation group. Each capitation group might only have enough funding for one patient to receive the transplant, unless basic services were cut for everyone else in that group. This example shows that such a system would be unfair, not simply the unfortunate result of a social lottery.[16] A decision has been made on a system-wide basis to distribute goods so that the total system will do less than it can afford to for its members.

RESTRICTIVE GATEKEEPING: COUNTERARGUMENTS AND REBUTTAL

Many now argue that, despite the problems outlined here, the rising cost of health care would be best-controlled by plans that assign a restrictive gatekeeping role to the physician. This argument has been advanced in several ways, each of which will be critiqued.

De Facto Gatekeeping

Some argue that physicians have always practiced for profit,[17] and are already de facto (actual) gatekeepers. Because physicians are the ones who actually control the supply and can influence the demand for medical interventions, cost-saving mechanisms might, therefore, be efficiently designed to control the behavior of physicians by linking physician income to decreased use of tests and therapies.

Some would further note that, in a fee-for-service system, the physician already has an incentive to be a factitious gatekeeper (that is, to order unnecessary tests and treatments in order to generate profit). This practice is clearly morally reprehensible and is not openly advocated, but is nonetheless a real phenomenon. It is alleged that the only important difference between a restrictive gatekeeping system, with financial incentives for limiting services, and a fee-for-service system is that the former encourages cost control, not cost escalation. The two systems are otherwise considered morally equivalent.

But restrictive gatekeeping is not just fee-for-service spelled backwards. The differences between the two systems are not symmetric. First, in fee-for-service, the interests of patients are generally congruent with the interests of physicians. Those physicians who exceed the bounds within which these interests coincide (that is, those who practice factitious gatekeeping) are condemned by society.[18] If such behavior reaches the level of fraud, these physicians may be subject to civil or even criminal charges. In contrast, when financial incentives are provided for cost control, patient interest is opposed to physician interest across the entire spectrum of diagnosis and treatment. Each step taken to help the patient can hurt the physician. Restrictive gatekeeping thus requires more moral strength than is expected by a fee-for-service system, in which failures of character are, sadly, already all too common. Also, because utilization review has not been extremely successful in controlling overuse, one must wonder whether such review will be sufficient to protect patients against underuse.

A second reason that fee for service and restrictive gatekeeping are asymmetric becomes apparent when one examines the system from the perspective of the patient. All systems are imperfect. The most important question may be, where does society want the margin of error to lie? Suppose, for example, that a patient with leukemia needed a computerized tomographic scan of the head and that, ideally, only one such scan was indicated. One suspects that most patients would, if given the choice of imperfect systems, prefer a system in which the margin of error was shaded toward overuse (so that they might receive a second scan of marginal utility) to one in which the margin of error was shaded toward underuse (so that they might not receive any scan at all). This example is not intended as a defense of a fee-for-service system, nor is it in any sense a defense of overutilization. These comments are, instead, a caution that restrictive gatekeeping may introduce more problems than it corrects.

Third, not all overuse of medical technology is driven by physicians' desire for profit, and it is not clear how much overuse would be curtailed in a system of restrictive gatekeeping. Much of the overuse is generated by inadequate medical thinking – the hasty and thoughtless ordering of tests. For example, overuse is clearly a problem even in university hospitals, where physicians are salaried and do not personally profit from the overuse. The love affair that American physicians and patients have with technology and a fear of malpractice suits also contribute to the overuse of resources. The problem is not simply one of controlling physician greed.

Finally, one should note that a fee-for-service system is not the only alternative to restrictive gatekeeping. The choice before society is not simply one of fee-for-service or restrictive gatekeeping. For example, salaried positions, while imperfect, have certain clear advantages. They can prevent factitious gatekeeping without introducing the problems of restrictive gatekeeping. They eliminate the incentive to test or treat only for profit. Of course, the widespread implementation of salary systems alone will not eliminate the overuse of technology, which is also driven by physician intolerance of uncertainty or by the practice of defensive medicine. But these latter problems would be better addressed through the reform of medical education and reform of the tort system. Such an effort would be an attempt to fix medicine by reforming the profession and the society, rather than an attempt to control the poor performance of the profession by appealing to the vices of physicians.

Clearly, salary systems may also generate different problems. They may, for example, provide a financial disincentive for physicians to put personal effort into the care of patients, or may lead to increased use of technology simply because it requires less effort. Given the alternatives, however, the combination of a program of intensive physician education with the enactment of tort reform and the introduction of a salary system (which U.S. physicians have accepted as the norm for housestaff and faculty in university hospitals, and which has served the public well for years), seems to be a viable and morally preferable option.

Autonomy

Proponents of restrictive gatekeeping argue that if costs must be controlled, a strategy of restrictive gatekeeping gives greater freedom to physicians and patients than do other cost-control strategies. No particular test or therapy is ruled out completely. Restrictive gatekeeping provides a softer way to say no. The "unseen hand" of market forces can assume responsibility for denying services. Costs will be cut because physicians will naturally come to a break-point at which delivery of health care and their own personal income needs have been met.

It is incorrect, however, to conclude that such a system would provide more freedom than plans that categorically ration care. Imagine that one has signed up for a college meal plan in which one pays a set fee for all one's meals for a year. Imagine that the boss has told the staff that they can serve anything that anyone needs or wants, but that as soon as staff expenditures exceed a certain amount, staff salaries will be cut. The cooks must "work out the details" for the students. The purported freedom of the practitioners and patients in a system of restrictive gatekeeping is analogous to the freedom of these cooks and hungry students. If the management has decided to budget only enough money for beans for everyone, the cooks can serve the patrons a variety of beans but nothing else, unless the cooks pay for it themselves, or unless the students bribe them, or unless the cooks decide that some students deserve steak while others deserve starvation. This system seems to provide an extremely limited form of autonomy, and is no more free than a system in which the management simply announces that they can only afford to buy and serve beans. At least the students would then know with whom they had to argue if they wanted a change.

Autonomy is exercised most fully in an environment characterized by equality and knowledge. In an HMO, autonomy requires, at the least, complete disclosure regarding coverage limitations and a genuine informed consent at the time patients join.[11] In a representative democracy, autonomy requires significant citizen participation in the decision-making process regarding cost control. These decisions should not be made solely by physicians or third-party payers.

Less Bureaucracy

Proponents of the restrictive gatekeeper role for physicians can also make the claim that their system would be less bureaucratically burdensome for doctors and patients. There would be no need for either elaborate government monitoring or for cumbersome agencies to make funding decisions. Market forces would "naturally" shape distribution.

Indeed, restrictive gatekeeping might be a very efficient system for controlling costs. It might require a less bureaucratic decision-making structure than would a system in which the public joined the profession in deciding what diagnostic and treatment modalities were to be limited. But it is not impossible a priori to conceive of an efficient system of public decision-making for health care rationing. Efficiency alone is an insufficient moral argument.

Some have also argued that actual individual cases vary far too widely to be subjected to categorical rationing procedures. Rationing decisions, they argue, are therefore most efficiently made by individual physicians treating individual patients, respecting the variability inherent in individuals and diseases.[12] Decisions to make certain modalities of treatment universally unavailable, however, do not detract from the recognition of the variability inherent in individual cases. Western physicians working in Third-World countries are aware of profound limitations on what they can provide, yet they render in good conscience the best care they can from the little they have for the good of each patient, as the case dictates, and often with great efficiency.

The Iatrogenic Burden

Finally, although medical care has certainly achieved great success in the 20th century, this has frequently been only a qualified success. Medical care brings with it untold side-effects, partial successes, and burdens for many of the patients it serves. It can be argued that by making physicians think twice about ordering tests and treatments, restrictive gatekeeping will save not only money but will also save patient lives, and will reduce the burden of iatrogenic illness.

Iatrogenic disease is, obviously, a real concern for both doctors and patients. Given the moral problems associated with restrictive gatekeeping, however, it seems that the problem of iatrogenic disease, whether due to errors of commission or errors of omission, would be better addressed by other means. The profession might shift its research efforts to put greater emphasis on the development of less toxic and dangerous therapies, and to develop more effective programs of peer review and continuing medical education. The government might also help by enacting genuine tort reform as part of an effort to stop the practice of defensive medicine.

CONCLUSION

There is much to reform in American medicine, but the cause of health care reform will not be advanced if attempts to reform the structure of health care financing are deleterious to the moral underpinnings of the medical enterprise. Cost-control efforts that place the physician either in the role of unilateral bedside rationer or restrictive gatekeeper threaten the integrity of medicine as a profession. Issues of cost control must be seen in the context both of other issues in health care delivery and in the broader social context of a nation that needs to recover a sense of virtue and of citizenship.[19] In this context, it seems preferable to begin the effort at cost control in medicine by reforming the profession, rather than by appealing to the vices of a profession that might yet have a chance to credibly claim to be noble.

APPENDIX: DEFINITION OF TERMS

The following definitions, largely adapted from the work of Pellegrino,[20] have been used in this discussion:

Cost Control

Any and all methods that are used to help decrease the level of health care expenditure are called cost-control measures. This very broad term is used to cover anything from educational efforts designed to teach physicians to be more cost-effective in their use of resources to a policy of explicitly denying life-saving therapies to patients to conserve resources.

Rationing

Health care rationing is taken here to mean an intentional plan to limit the distribution of indicated services and goods, motivated by the perception that supplies are scarce. Indicated services and goods are those which are effective in furthering the traditional goals of medicine: to cure, to relieve, or to comfort the sick. This definition would exclude futile services, such as treating viral upper respiratory infections with penicillin, or superfluous services, such as cosmetic surgery, which do not correct diseases, injuries or postsurgical defects. The perception that supplies are scarce might arise from allocational decisions made by others, by natural scarcity, by misperceptions, or by any combination of these factors. Thus, rationing is considered to be a particular form of cost control.

(Others would define rationing more broadly so that it would include "implicit rationing" – the sum of all practices and decisions which limit the supply or accessibility of medical goods and services. As a stipulative definition, this is not wrong. It seems extremely broad, however, and a less-than-optimal use of language. Under such a definition, for example, the with-holding of tube feedings from Nancy Cruzan would be accounted rationing. This would seem to obscure the issues at stake in this discussion.)

De Facto Gatekeeping

The physician is the sole source of entry into the contemporary medical system – the one who orders the tests and prescribes the treatments and arranges the consultations. The physician has an inherent obligation, in the interest of the patient, to use only those tests and treatments which are medically indicated. It is in this sense that the physician is a de facto gatekeeper. While the legitimacy of this role has been contested (21), most persons, regardless of their ethical viewpoint, accept this role as a starting point, and do not see it as morally problematic per se that the physician is the keeper of contemporary medical knowledge and power.

Restrictive Gatekeeping

Any system in which either the physician's income or the money available to the physicians to provide care for other patients is tied to the physician's proficiency in limiting tests, treatments and consultations ordered for patients. This method is often used, for example, in a for-profit HMO. It can take several forms, for example, financial penalties for the use of resources at a level deemed to be excessive, financial rewards (such as bonuses) for the use of resources at a level deemed to be efficient, or those capitation systems in which a fixed amount of money is allotted to the physician to use in caring for a fixed number of patients over a determined period.

Fee-for-Service

This model refers to the traditional system in which physician income is directly proportional to the billing generated by services rendered to patients. This billing process has now come to be largely mediated by third-party payers, but remains essentially intact. In a fee-for-service model, no capitation is provided to individual physicians or physician groups, and no personal financial incentives encourage physicians to limit care.

Factitious Gatekeeping

In a fee-for-service system, the physician may order unnecessary tests, treatments or consultations purely for personal or corporate profit. This practice is called factitious gatekeeping.

Salary

Salary systems are taken to include all systems in which the physician's income is determined by time (for example, annually or hourly). In salary systems, neither physician income nor the budget available to care for patients depends upon proficiency in limiting per capita patient care expenditures. Salary systems are often used, for example, in teaching hospitals.

KEY IDEAS IN THIS ARTICLE:

- Bedside rationing and restrictive gatekeeping (i.e., the use of financial incentives) are morally unacceptable roles for physicians.

- Rationing is unacceptable because it is often unnecessary and tends to be idiosyncratic, arbitrary, discriminatory, and unlikely to result in the desired redistribution of funds.

- Restrictive gatekeeping is unacceptable for several reasons. First, it enables administrators (the real decision-makers) to shirk their responsibility to inform the public about which services will and will not be covered. Second, although it seems preferable to have those at the bedside adjust the distribution of benefits to individual patients, this ends up being inequitable. It would be preferable to withhold a class of technology from everyone rather than make it available to some patients and not to others. How does one choose fairly and consistently among those who might benefit? Third, restrictive gatekeeping is based on physician self-interest, and this conflicts with and undermines the traditional expectation of altruism; such a conflict creates moral distress for physicians. Fourth, the use of financial incentives further erodes an already declining sense of trust between physicians and patients; it will weaken the doctor-patient relationship.

- If rationing is essential to contain costs, a morally preferable approach would be one that applies equally to all members of society, and which rations by classes of technology which have been decided upon after open, public debate by identifiable individuals who are clearly responsible to society.

- A salary system for physicians (along with tort reform) is morally preferable to restrictive gatekeeping.

A SUGGESTED PROCESS FOR REFLECTING ON THIS ARTICLE:

(See pages 234-254 for other processes that might better fit your goals and objectives.)

1. Rationing is unnecessary in order to control healthcare costs.
   ☐ strongly agree ☐ agree ☐ ? ☐ disagree ☐ strongly disagree
   Comment:

2. Bedside rationing is idiosyncratic, arbitrary, discriminatory, unlikely to result in the desired redistribution of funds and is, therefore, unethical.
   ☐ strongly agree ☐ agree ☐ ? ☐ disagree ☐ strongly disagree
   Comment:

3. Restrictive gatekeeping enables administrators to shirk their responsibility to inform the public about which services will and will not be covered.

◻ strongly agree ◻ agree ◻ ? ◻ disagree ◻ strongly disagree
Comment:

4. It would be preferable to withhold a class of technology from everyone rather than make it available to some and not to others.
   ◻ strongly agree ◻ agree ◻ ? ◻ disagree ◻ strongly disagree
   Comment:

5. Restrictive gatekeeping is based on physician self-interest, and this conflicts with and undermines the traditional expectation of altruism.
   ◻ strongly agree ◻ agree ◻ ? ◻ disagree ◻ strongly disagree
   Comment:

6. Rationing should only occur after open, public debate by identifiable individuals who are clearly responsible to society.
   ◻ strongly agree ◻ agree ◻ ? ◻ disagree ◻ strongly disagree
   Comment:

7. Is rationing occurring in your institution? If so, where and by whom? How are these decisions being made? Is this method ethically acceptable? Why? Why not?

8. Does your institution/organization have any ethical standards to guide rationing decisions? If not, why not? Should there be? How might that occur? If so, what are they? Do they work?

9. If rationing is occurring in your institution/organization, is anyone following the impact of rationing decisions on patients?

ENDNOTES

1. Office of National Cost Estimates. *Health care financing review.* 1990; 11:1.

2. Rich S. Health costs to consume 16% of GNP by 2000, agency says. *Washington Post.* Sat., Aug. 24, 1991:A2.

3. Wennberg JE. Outcomes research, cost-containment, and the fear of health care rationing. *N Engl J Med* 1990;323:1202-4.

4. Menzel PT. *Strong Medicine: The Ethical Rationing of Health Care.* New York: Oxford University Press; 1990.

5. Aaron H, Schwartz WB. Rationing health care: The choice before us. *Science.* 1990;247: 418-22.

6. Callahan D. Rationing medical progress: The way to affordable health care. *N Engl J Med* 1990;322:1810-3.

7. Pellegrino ED, Thomasma DC. For the Patient's Good: The Restoration of Beneficence in Health Care. New York: Oxford University Press; 1988:172-89.

8. Relman AS. Is rationing inevitable? *N Eng J Med* 1990;322:1809-10.

9. Pellegrino ED, Thomasma DC. For the Patient's Good: The Restoration of Beneficence in Health Care. New York: Oxford University Press; 1988:54-55.

10. Aristotle. Nichomachean Ethics. 1131a.21-24. T Irwin, trans. Indianapolis, Indiana: Hackett; 1985:123.

11. Levinson DF. Towards full disclosure of referral restrictions and financial incentives by prepaid health plans. *N Engl J Med* 1987, 317:1729-31.

12. Welch HG. Should the health care forest be selectively thinned by physicians or clear cut by payers? *Ann Intern Med.* 1991;115:223-6.

13. Flexner A. Is social work a profession? *School and Society.* 1915; 1:901-11.

14. Mackie DL, Decker DK. *Group and IPA HMOs.* Rockville, Maryland: Aspen Systems; 1981:155-6, 165-6.

15. Welch WP, Hillman AL, Pauly MV. Toward new typologies for HMOs. *Milband Q.* 1990;68:221-43.

16. Englehardt HT. *The foundations of bioethics.* New York: Oxford University Press; 1986:342-3.

17. Rie MA, Engelhardt HT. Morality for the medical-industrial complex. *N Eng J Med* 1988;319:108-69.

18. Shaw GB. The doctor's dilemma. In: *Bernard Shaw: The Complete Plays and Prefaces.* vol. I. New York: Dodd, Mead, and Co.; 1962:1-188.

19. Bellah RN, Masden R, Sullivan WM, Swidler A, Tipton SM. *Habits of the Heart: Individualism and Commitment in American Life.* Berkeley, California: University of California Press; 1985,

20. Pellegrino ED. Rationing health care: the ethics of moral gatekeeping. *Journal of Contemporary Health Law Policy.* 1986;2:23-45.

21. Illich I. Medical Nemesis. New York: Bantam Books; 1976,

Chapter 15

The Unbearable Rightness of Bedside Rationing:
Physician Duties in a Climate of Cost Containment

Peter A. Ubel, MD, Robert M. Arnold, MD

A LOCAL INTERNIST IS IN THE PROCESS OF ORDERING AN INTRAVENOUS PYELOGRAM for a patient she suspects of having kidney problems, when a medical student shadowing her in clinic interrupts. The student wants to know why the physician is not ordering a low-osmolality contrast agent for the patient, having read that they are less likely to cause serious side-effects than high-osmolality contrast agents. The physician realizes that the medical student is correct, but rejects the suggestion, telling the student that "low-osmolality contrast agents are the standard of care for low-risk patients."

The physician is uneasy about her response to the medical student. She was taught that physicians ought to pursue their patients' best interests, regardless of cost. According to this teaching, it is wrong for physicians to ration at the bedside. Yet now she realizes that there is only one reason to order a high- instead of a low-osmolality contrast agent for this patient: the high-osmolality contrast agent is cheaper![1-3] Despite this realization, she is still unwilling to pursue the marginal benefits that could be gained with a low-osmolality contrast agent, believing that they are not worth the extra price.

Physicians, like this one, are increasingly under pressure to serve two masters. On one hand, they have been taught to do what they can to promote their patients' best interests. On the other hand, they face great pressure from the government, third-party payers, and the general public to serve societal interests by containing health care costs.

Political and social forces are likely to exacerbate these pressures. Those politicians attempting to reform the health care system have promised that they will meet the contradictory goals of containing health care costs and increasing the number of people with adequate health care coverage. Meanwhile, prepaid health care plans proliferate, advertising low costs and seemingly unrestricted benefits to prospective patients. Neither group wants to acknowledge the need to ration care. Thus, the easiest solution may be for politicians and third-party payers to avoid explicit acknowledgment of the need to ration, while creating policies that implicitly require physicians to ration at the bedside.

A number of physicians and ethicists have argued that, despite these pressures, physicians should never ration at the bedside.[4-11] In this article, we look at several mechanisms available to governments and third-party payers that, when used alone or in combination, could potentially help control health care spending. We argue that for any combination of these mechanisms to succeed, they must be able to control costs without causing undue harm to patient care. We conclude that, at present, none of these mechanisms will be able to successfully control costs unless physicians relax their advocacy roles. Although bedside rationing raises serious moral problems, these are outweighed by the important social goal of containing health care costs, while providing adequate health care to those who need it. At least for the short and medium term, bedside rationing will be a necessary component of any successful cost-containment strategy.

In this article, we use the term *bedside rationing* to refer to physicians' actions to withhold beneficial care from patients that the physicians were free to offer to them. As we use the term, it refers mainly to rationing that is done either without patients being aware of the rationing or, less often, with patients being aware but being given no choice. We will not concern ourselves with instances where physicians talk patients into accepting rationing.

The traditional view of physicians' duties holds that because of the moral problems raised by bedside rationing, physicians should never ration at the bedside.[4-7,10,12,13] This view does not require physicians to ignore all concerns other than their patients' best interests. For example, it allows physicians to balance their patients' interests with their family's well-being, and even requires physicians to relax their strict advocacy of patient confidentiality when it conflicts with more important public health needs. But the traditional view does require physicians to ignore the financial interests of society when they are making clinical decisions. Under this view, it is never morally acceptable for physicians to ration at the bedside.

There are several justifications for the traditional view, some stronger than others. First, some authors argue that bedside rationing is wrong because it takes away beneficial services from patients when, instead, rising health care costs should be controlled through the elimination of waste.[5,14] According to this view, bedside rationing is wrong because any type of rationing is wrong. This view ignores several unique features of the health care industry that make it unlikely that we can control costs solely through the elimination of waste. Health care is highly labor-intensive; thus, it is less amenable to increased productivity than are things like the manufacturing industry. Thus, many health care costs will continue to rise relative to other parts of the economy. In addition, new technology does not lower the price of goods in the health care industry like it does in other industries. In fact, much of the rise in health care expenditures is the result of new technologies.[15-17] This makes "waste elimination," at best, a one-shot savings, soon to be outstripped by other inflationary forces. While we ought to do what we can to eliminate waste, we cannot expect to control health care costs without some type of rationing.

Second, some authors argue that bedside rationing is wrong because it creates savings that are not guaranteed to benefit other patients.[18,19] We cannot know, for example, whether the money saved on a low-yield diagnostic test will be used to provide more beneficial health care goods, such as childhood vaccines or prenatal care. The savings may, instead, go toward other health services that bring no more benefit or, worse yet, toward insurance company profits. However, we are unconvinced by this argument because it incorrectly assumes that bedside rationing is unjust unless money saved on one patient is guaranteed to bring greater medical benefit to other patients. The rise in medical expenses in recent years, combined with other government activities, has put our country in a position where health care dollars are competing with other important social goals for funding.[20] As the government debates how much to cut welfare, education, and other social programs, it becomes implausible to say that money saved at the bedside should not go toward other important societal goals. We take too narrow a view of justice when we forbid physicians from rationing marginally beneficial services at the same time that the government cannot pay its bills, small businesses cannot afford health insurance for their employees, and large businesses struggle to compete with foreign companies that have lower medical costs. There is no morally compelling reason to argue that money saved on one health care service must go toward other health care services.

We are equally unconvinced by a more limited criticism of bedside rationing: that physicians should not ration unless they can guarantee that the savings will bring more benefit (medical *or nonmedical*) to other people. While this view would allow physicians to ration at the bedside if they could guarantee that the money would go toward crime prevention or some other laudable goal, it would not allow them to ration if the money might go toward VCRs, earrings or tennis racquets. The problem with this view is that, for some patients. having a VCR is more important than having certain medical services. For example, many people would undoubtedly prefer owning a VCR to spending a similar amount of money on a screening test with a one-in-a-million chance of benefiting them. Because these choices are so complicated, we must rely on our present, and imperfect, political process to decide how to divide resources among the many ways people would like to spend them. Any theory of justice needs to figure out how to balance the rights of individuals to spend their wealth on themselves with the need to assure some amount of basic social systems that all can enjoy, regardless of their ability to pay. In our present social system, we tax people in order to guarantee certain services, while allowing people to spend the rest of their wealth largely as they see fit. Whether we should spend less money on VCRs and more on health care is a question for our society to answer through legislation, union negotiations over insurance coverage, etc. And the consensus from these corners is that we spend too much on health care relative to other social goods. Thus, we must look for ways, including bedside rationing, that will limit how much we spend on marginally beneficial health care services.

Third, bedside rationing is criticized for being vulnerable to discrimination. If physicians are told that it is acceptable to ration at the bedside, they may disproportionately withhold services from patients of certain races or socioeconomic groups. Similarly, bedside rationing is prone to random variability which, while not necessarily discriminatory, still raises serious ethical concerns.[8-10] For example, some physicians will be more likely than others to withhold marginally beneficial care from their patients. This leaves patients in a situation where their choice of physicians affects whether or not they get certain marginally beneficial services. Those aware of this variability will be at an advantage, because they can be more aggressive about obtaining marginally beneficial services.

This is a more convincing criticism of bedside rationing. Indeed, whatever forms of rationing we use, we ought to be aware of the potential for discrimination. Thus, for example, rationing according to ability, to pay discriminates against people with less money. Rationing according to disease state discriminates against people with certain diseases. Regardless of how we choose to ration care, discrimination against socially stigmatized or less powerful groups is likely to occur. Even in the Veterans Administration Medical Centers, devoid as they are of any incentive to treat one patient ahead of another, research has raised questions about whether blacks receive the same intensity of services as whites.[21] We need data to tell us how much discrimination to expect in systems that rely on bedside rationing to control costs vs. ones that do not. The possibility that discrimination will be aggravated by bedside rationing must be taken seriously, and to the extent that this occurs, we ought to rely as little as possible on bedside rationing.

Fourth, bedside rationing is opposed by those who believe that it will adversely affect the doctor-patient relationship.[6,10] According to this view, if patients find out that physicians are not giving them access to potentially beneficial services, they may lose trust in them. This, too, is a serious problem with bedside rationing. However, it is not so serious that it should preclude physicians from ever rationing at the bedside. There are no data to either back up or refute the claim that bedside rationing will damage the doctor-patient relationship. We have little idea what patients think of bedside rationing vs. other types of rationing schemes. For all we know, patients may accept some amount of bedside rationing if they think it is the best way to control costs. In fact, given the amount of bedside rationing that physicians do everyday,[22] it seems that we would have already seen more evidence of its damaging effects on the doctor-patient relationship. In addition, the effects of bedside rationing on the doctor-patient relationship are likely to be limited because patients often will not be aware that care is being rationed. It is likely that most instances of bedside rationing are too subtle for many patients to pick up on. A physician orders a diagnostic test with 90% sensitivity, instead of a much more expensive one with 91% sensitivity. While some physicians may worry that this raises legal risks about failing to provide informed consent to patients,[23] others argue that the law has not left us with any other options, since most cost-control measures have been limited by physicians' legal efforts to maintain their professional autonomy.[24]

We do not mean to argue that lack of evidence of damage proves that there is no damage. Indeed, it is crucial to perform research to see how patients react to physicians' rationing decisions. But it is also crucial to be open-minded to the plausible possibility that patients will not react negatively to physicians who ration marginally beneficial care. Because we have so little data about bedside rationing's consequences, we must be cautious about accepting consequentialistic arguments put forth by its opponents. The problems raised by bedside rationing, while serious, are not devastating. Thus, before we abandon any thought of bedside rationing, we need to examine its alternatives more closely.

AN EVALUATION OF SOME ALTERNATIVES TO BEDSIDE RATIONING

A number of cost-control mechanisms are already in use that attempt to control costs without relying on bedside rationing. In general, these cost-control mechanisms rely on rules and procedures to ration care, allowing physicians to pursue their patients' best interests as far as the rules allow them. For example, formulary committees limit the medicines that physicians can prescribe for hospitalized patients.[25] Utilization reviewers check to see whether or not particular patients require ongoing hospitalization.[24] Governments administer Certificate of Need laws to limit the amount of expensive new technology available to physicians and their patients,[26] and practice guidelines are developed to encourage physicians to practice more cost-effective medicine.[27]

It is crucial to understand what we mean when we say that these mechanisms do not rely on bedside rationizing to control costs. Suppose two medications exist to treat a condition, and one is slightly better than the other but costs much more. If a hospital formulary committee decides not to allow physicians to offer the more-expensive drug, then the formulary committee has made a rationing decision. By making the rationing decision at this level, the committee has removed the need for physicians to ration this medication at the bedside. In this example, physicians on the formulary committee who support the decision are involved in rationing at the committee level,[25] but they are not involved in bedside rationing. And physicians treating patients at the bedside, no longer allowed to offer the better medication, are not making rationing decisions at all, but are merely complying with the rationing decisions made by the formulary committee. In this manner, rationing decisions made at the level of a formulary committee reduce the need for physicians to ration at the bedside.

There are other ways to control health care costs that do not rely on bedside rationing. Consider, for example, the state of Oregon's plan to provide Medicaid funds for a limited number of health care services, excluding those it thinks offer the least amount of benefit.[28-30] This plan attempts to control health care costs by narrowing the number of treatments that physicians will get paid to perform. In essence, it puts physicians into a position where, even if they think a patient might benefit from a certain treatment, they will not get reimbursed if they offer it. Like a formulary committee, the Oregon plan relieves physicians of the need to ration at the bedside by setting strict limits on what physicians will be reimbursed to do.

For any of these mechanisms to succeed without relying on bedside rationing, the rationing decisions made through them must be enforceable. If formulary committee decisions are only understood as recommendations, then physicians holding the traditional view of physician duties will be morally obligated to ignore them whenever a drug not recommended by the formulary committee is more beneficial. Thus, for example, if a formulary committee recommends use of streptokinase in patients with acute myocardial infarction, physicians who think tissue plasminogen activator is a better drug should use it, despite its cost.[22]

Can these mechanisms control costs successfully without relying on bedside rationing? Experience has shown that formulary committees, utilization reviewers and practice guidelines may not control health care costs. Formulary committees have saved money in some areas and have increased costs in others.[31] Utilization review and Certificate of Need laws have been weakened by loopholes and "physician gaming."[32] And practice guidelines have largely been ignored by physicians, who either do not learn about them or do not believe them.[33-36] Improving physicians' knowledge of and compliance with rules will cost money. We do not yet know whether this will be made up by the savings they bring.[37] In short, it is not certain that any of these methods can, or will contain health care costs without relying on some amount of bedside rationing.

Let us assume, for the sake of argument, that these mechanisms, alone or in combination, could circumscribe physicians' actions well enough to control cost without relying on physicians to ration at the bedside. How complex would this circumscription have to be to successfully control costs? The circumscription could, theoretically, take as "simple" a form as Oregon's plan to ration Medicaid services. Its rationing plan, while no small task to create, lumps all health care services into fewer than 700 "condition-treatment pairs." Physicians are paid or not paid to treat patients depending on whether their conditions fall under Oregon's list of reimbursable condition-treatment pairs.

This degree of simplicity comes at a cost: it is unlikely to capture the subtleties of clinical practice. For example, under Oregon's plan, physicians are not reimbursed to treat sarcoidosis.[38] In choosing not to pay for treatment of this illness, Oregon determined that because sarcoidosis often remits spontaneously, it was less beneficial to treat than other conditions that it chose to cover. This in no way implies that medical treatment of patients with sarcoidosis never brings substantial benefit or that physicians could not identify such patients. In fact, there are some patients who gain great benefit from treatment of sarcoidosis. Instead, because Oregon could not fit such subtleties into a list of 700 health services, it had to decide which services offered the most benefit, even if that meant cutting out some people who could gain from treatment.

This points out a crucial aspect of any kind of health care reform that tries to eliminate the need for physicians to relax their advocacy duties. The system must contain enough detail and complexity to adequately circumscribe physicians' actions; otherwise, physicians holding the traditional view will interpret the rules in ways that benefit their patients, even at great cost to society. In addition, the rules need to retain enough flexibility to capture the subtleties of clinical practice; otherwise, the rules will harm patients who do not fit them well. Creating such rules is an enormous task. Exciting work is being done to develop and implement practice guidelines for everything from acute chest pain[39] to ankle sprains.[40] Eventually, such guidelines may be able to capture the subtleties of clinical practice. But no immediate health care reforms will be able to rely on a successful stable of such rules and guidelines.

EVALUATING COST-CONTROL MECHANISMS THAT RELY, AT LEAST IN PART, ON BEDSIDE RATIONING

Some mechanisms control costs by strictly circumscribing physicians' actions; others control costs by setting flexible goals for physicians so they can retain control of individual clinical decisions. These mechanisms attempt to influence physicians' aggregate utilization patterns without stating when the physicians can or cannot obtain things like ankle films. For example, a system could control costs by setting global budgets or by setting spending targets for individual physicians. This system would not need to dictate clinical care to physicians. Physicians in such systems would not need to be monitored to see if they complied with elaborate practice guidelines or reimbursement rules. Rather, they could be monitored to see if they met some kind of standard for average expenditures. In meeting those standards, physicians could decide when a potential benefit was worth seeking for their patients, perhaps on occasion offering services that may not be recommended in practice guidelines, and perhaps on other occasions withholding marginal benefits that they do not think justify the expense.

It is important to understand that this type of system is not necessarily devoid of rules. Utilization reviews, formulary committees and the like may play a role in containing costs. But the rules used in this type of system will not be expected to carry the entire burden of cost containment. Instead, physicians will be allowed, perhaps even expected, to ration marginally beneficial care at the bedside. This will allow health care plans to develop rules that are more flexible and more appropriate to the complexities of clinical practice.[41,42] Consequently, the plans will be likely to result in better patient care.

The tradeoff, thus, is clear. Without bedside rationing, we can only contain costs with a complex set of rules circumscribing physicians' actions, rules that are likely to have patients whose specific medical conditions are not adequately captured by the rules, With bedside rationing, we can contain costs with less complex rules, but we must also worry that the discretion this gives physicians will be used discriminatorily or will harm the doctor-patient relationship. What should we do?

THE SHORT- AND MEDIUM-RUN ANSWER

In the long run, it is not clear which of these mechanisms we should use. It is conceivable that we could devise rules and procedures that remove physicians from the need to make individualized rationing decisions, while preserving a high standard of clinical practice.[43] In this case, there would be no reason to ration at the bedside. On the other hand, it is also conceivable that no set of rules will control costs without seriously damaging the quality of patient care. Clinical medicine is a science of particulars, so even the most rigorous guidelines may not capture everything they need to. In this latter case, we will be left with a tradeoff between relying exclusively on rules to ration (while reducing the quality of patient care) or relying in part on physicians to ration (while creating the possibility that they will not do so in a fair manner).

In the short run, and probably in the medium run of the next 5 to 10 years, the moral choice is much clearer: we are in no position to eliminate bedside rationing. First, if physicians were told they could no longer ration at the bedside, the cost of health care would continue to rise even faster than it already is. While few investigators have studied the actual incidence of bedside rationing,[22] and no one that we know of has determined its economic impact, our clinical experience and our conversations with other physicians suggest that the practice is widespread. Physicians ration so often they do not even realize it. They order computarized tomographic scans, even though magnetic resonance imaging may yield a fraction more benefit; they prescribe Benadryl, even though Seldane has fewer side-effects; and they adjust the frequency of screening pap smears when the yield of more frequent screening becomes too small to be worth it. All these actions essentially save money by rationing small benefits from patients.

Second, we have not developed enough guidelines and rationing rules to effectively contain costs. As mentioned above, Oregon has made the most serious attempt to set up an administrative rationing mechanism that will remove the need for bedside rationing. But it is too early to know whether its system can control costs. Many of the categories of covered services include generous room for physician interpretation, stating, for example, that the cost of certain cancer therapies will be reimbursed if the cancer is "treatable."[30] Physicians clinging to the traditional view of their duties could interpret this type of language in ways that will undermine Oregon's efforts to control costs.

Third, and most importantly, the ability of rules to contain costs is dependent on physicians' willingness to accept rationing. If physicians feel that their duty is to do everything within their power to benefit patients, they will find ways around all but the most stringent rules.[32] Some of us may counter that physicians who follow the spirit of the rules will not undermine their effectiveness. But the spirit of many of these rules results in rationing marginally beneficial services from patients. If that is the spirit that opponents of bedside rationing want physicians to accept, then we have a distinction without a difference, for we have accepted the notion that physicians ought to restrain their advocacy roles, if only enough to withhold marginal benefits that cost society large sums of money.

AN (AT LEAST TEMPORARY) ETHIC OF BEDSIDE RATIONING

Because physicians will be required to do some amount of bedside rationing for at least the short and medium-term, we must begin to define those factors that physicians should consider in deciding when it is appropriate to ration at the bedside.

The moral acceptability of bedside rationing depends crucially on which services physicians think to ration. For bedside rationing to be morally tolerable, physicians should base rationing decisions on medical costs and benefits, not on racial or sexual biases. In addition, they should only ration marginally beneficial services, not ones that bring significant benefits to their patients. We have been using the term *marginally beneficial* throughout this article to describe the types of services physicians could, most plausibly, be allowed to ration. Defining this term precisely is impossible. But several concepts can help to clarify what it means in a way that can begin to settle the moral debate.

First, similar to the way we measure cost-effectiveness, physicians should think of marginally beneficial services in terms of both a numerator (costs) and a denominator (benefits). We need to know something about both before we can judge a service. Very inexpensive services, such as a screening calcium test, may offer minuscule benefits that do not justify their cost. Similarly, extremely expensive services may offer significant benefits that more than justify their cost. Oregon ignored this insight when, before developing the Medicaid plan discussed above, it decided to curtail funding for all transplants, figuring it could use the funds in more beneficial ways.[44] Its decision, ultimately repealed, concentrated only on the cost of transplantation, and thus overlooked other services which, when both cost and benefit were measured, would have proved to be a worse use of state money.

Second, the true cost-effectiveness of a health care intervention can only be determined if something is known about the costs and benefits of alternative interventions. For example, it would be wrong to determine the cost-effectiveness of a yearly pap smear by taking its costs and dividing by its benefits. This ignores the fact that most of the benefit of screening for cervical cancer can be achieved by screening every three years.[45] To calculate the cost-effectiveness of a yearly pap smear, one must first measure the extra cost of yearly pap smears as opposed to pap smears every three years, and then divide this by the extra benefit brought by yearly screening. From this point of view, one would have to spend more than $1 million for every year of life gained by yearly pap smears over every three years.[45]

Third, the cost-effectiveness of specific therapies often varies widely depending on patient preferences.[46] For example, the cost-effectiveness of radiation therapy for prostate cancer is greater for patients who place a high value on sexual potency than for those who do not.[47] Thus, physicians need to consider patients' preferences when they are making rationing choices. This includes finding out what the patients think about various outcomes that they may experience. It also includes talking about patients' out-of-pocket costs to find out, for example, whether they are willing to pay for the small benefits that they could receive with marginally beneficial services.

While the cost-effectiveness is a very helpful tool in making rationing decisions, it must be used with caution. The techniques used to measure cost and, especially, effectiveness do not necessarily reflect the relative value society places on various resources.[48] It is especially true when one is dealing with specific individuals who have potentially treatable illnesses. Society does not place a consistent value on people's lives.[49] It is willing to spend enormous sums of money to save one child who falls into a well, yet it is unwilling to spend the same amount to save more children through pre-natal care.[50] Physicians need to recognize this seeming inconsistency and factor that into their rationing decisions. Thus, physicians should be with-holding therapies from severely ill patients, even if cost-effectiveness studies suggest that there are better ways of spending health care dollars.

Physicians should not be expected to perform cost-effectiveness analyses at the bedside. Rather, they should become familiar enough with the concepts of cost-effectiveness so that they can more accurately identify marginally beneficial health care services. Indeed, given the necessity of bedside rationing, it is time to do more to train physicians in the economics of clinical decision-making.

CONCLUSIONS

While we have only begun to discuss how and when physicians should ration at the bedside, continuing this discussion is crucial for the future of medicine. Bedside rationing is here to stay, at least for the immediate future. It creates moral problems, but these have been overstated. In addition, those mechanisms that would control costs without relying on bedside rationing raise moral problems of their own, being too primitive at present to capture the subtleties of medical practice. For at least the next 5 to 10 years, physicians will need to ration at the bedside. The medical profession needs to admit this openly, so that physicians can begin to talk openly about when they ration, and so they can learn more about when they ought to ration. Physicians are less likely to find their dual roles (as patient and societal advocates) unbearable if they can talk together about how best to balance them.

The authors thank Baruch Brody, PhD. David MacPherson, MD, and Paula Greeno, MBA, for comments on earlier versions of this article. Reprint requests to Veterans Affairs Medical Center (111G.M.), University and Woodland avenues, Philadelphia, PA 19104 (Dr. Ubel).

KEY IDEAS IN THE ARTICLE:

- The moral problems associated with bedside rationing have been overstated and are outweighed by the important social goal of containing health care costs, while providing adequate health care to those who need it. In the absence of sufficient data concerning the negative consequences of bedside rationing, we should be cautious about rejecting it.

- The problems associated with bedside rationing are serious, but not overwhelming.

- For the short and medium-term, bedside rationing will be a necessary component of any successful cost-containment strategy.

- The alternatives to rationing – formulary committees, utilization review, certificates of need, practice guidelines and the like – have not been successful in controlling healthcare costs.

- Rationing should be made only on the basis of medical costs and benefits, and apply only to marginally beneficial services (i.e., services whose benefits do not justify their costs).

- A decision about whether or not to ration in the individual case would also need to consider the costs and benefits of alternative services, as well as what patients are willing to accept regarding outcomes.

A SUGGESTED PROCESS FOR REFLECTING ON THIS ARTICLE:

(See pages 234-254 for other processes that might better fit your goals and objectives.)

1. Bedside rationing by physicians is preferable to rationing by committees or administrators.
   ❐ strongly agree ❐ agree ❐ ? ❐ disagree ❐ strongly disagree
   Comment:

2. The potential ethical problems associated with bedside rationing are justified by the need to control health care costs.
   ❐ strongly agree ❐ agree ❐ ? ❐ disagree ❐ strongly disagree
   Comment:

3. Rationing should occur only on the basis of medical costs and benefits and apply only to marginally beneficial services.
   ❐ strongly agree ❐ agree ❐ ? ❐ disagree ❐ strongly disagree
   Comment:

4. Assume that rationing at the bedside is necessary. What guidelines would you propose to assist physicians in making those decisions? In developing these guidelines, keep in mind the ethical pitfalls associated with bedside rationing mentioned in the article. What ethical considerations shaped your principles?

Ethical Guidelines for Rationing	Ethical Considerations

ENDNOTES

1. Steinberg EP. Moore RD, Powe NR. et al. Safety and cost-effectiveness of high-osmolality as compared with low-osmolality contrast material in patients undergoing cardiac angiography. *N Engl J Med* 1992:326:425-430.

2. Eddy DM, Applying cost-effectiveness analysis: the inside story. *JAMA*. 1992:268:2575-2582.

3. Appel LJ., Steinberg EP, Powe NR, Anderson GF, Dwyer SA, Faden RR. Risk reduction from low osmolality contrast media: what do patients think it is worth? *Med Care*. 1990;28:324-337.

4. Abrams FR. Patient advocate or secret agent? *JAMA*. 1986;256:1784-1785.

5. Angell M. Cost containment and the physician. *JAMA*. 1985:254:1203-1207.

6. Hiatt HH. Protecting the medical commons. *N Engl J Med* 1975;293:235-241.

7. LaPuma J, Cassel CK, Humphrey H. Ethics, economics, and endocarditis: the physician's role in resource allocation. *Arch Intern Med*. 1988, 148:1809-1811.

8. Wolf SM. Health care reform and the future of physician ethics. *Hastings Cent Rep*. 1994;24:28-41.

9. Emanuel EJ, Brett AS. Managed competition and the patient-physician relationship. *N. Engl. J. Med*. 1993:329:879-882.

10. Sulmasy DP. Physicians, cost control, and ethics. *Ann Intern Med*. 1992;116:920-926.

11. American Medical Association Council on Ethical and Judicial Affairs. Ethical issues in managed care. *JAMA*. 1995;273:330-335.

12. Levinsky NG. The doctor's master. *N. Engl. J. Med*. 1984;311:1573-1575.

13. Brett AS, McCullough LB. When patients request specific interventions: defining the limits of the physician's obligation. *N. Engl. J. Med*. 1986; 315:1347-1351.

14. Brook RH, Lohr KN. Will we need to ration effective health care? *Issues Sci Technol*. Fall 1986: 68-77.

15. Aaron HJ, Schwartz WB. Rationing health care: the choice before us. *Science*. 1990;247:418-422.

16. Callahan D. Symbols, rationality, and justice: rationing health care. *Am J Law Med*. 1992;18:1-13.

17. Evans RW. Health care technology and the inevitability of resource allocation and rationing decisions. *JAMA*. 1983;249:2208-2219.

18. Daniels N. The ideal advocate and limited resources. *Theor Med*. 1987:8:69-80.

19. Cassel C. Doctors and allocation decisions: a new role in the new Medicare. *J Health Polit Policy Law* 1985:10:549-564.

20. Morreim EH. Fiscal scarcity and the inevitability of bedside budget balancing. *Arch Intern Med.* 1989:149:1012-1015.

21. Whittle J, Conigliaro J, Good CB, Lofgren R. Racial differences in the use of invasive cardiovascular procedures in the Department of Veterans Affairs medical system. *N. Engl. J. Med.* 1993; 329:621-627.

22. Brody B, Wray N, Barn S, Ashton C, Petersen N, Harward M. The impact of economic considerations on clinical decision making: the case of thrombolytic therapy. *Med Care.* 1991;29:899-910.

23. Miller FH. Denial of health care and informed consent in English and American law. *Am J Law Med.* 1992:18:37-71.

24. Hall M. Institutional control of physician behavior: legal barriers to health care cost containment. *Univ Pa Law Rev.* 1988:137:431-536.

25. Hochla PKO, Tuason VB. Pharmacy and therapeutics committee: cost-containment considerations. *Arch Intern Med,* 1992:152:1773-1775.

26. Furrow BR. The ethics of cost-containment: bureaucratic medicine and the doctor as patient-advocate. *J Law Ethics Public Policy.* 1988:3:187-225.

27. Brook RH. Practice guidelines and practicing medicine:are they compatible? *JAMA.* 1989;262: 3027-3030.

28. Fox DM, Leichter HM. Rationing care in Oregon: the new accountability. *Health Aff.* 1991;10:7-27.

29. Garland MJ. Rationing in public: Oregon's priority-setting methodology. In: Strosberg MA, Wiener JM, Baker R, Fein IA, eds. *Rationing America's Medical Care: The Oregon Plan and Beyond.* Washington. DC: Brookings Institution: 1992.

30. Oregon Health Services Commission. *Prioritization of Health Services: A Report to the Governor and Legislature.* Salem, Ore: Oregon Health Services Commission; December 4, 1992.

31. Sloan FA, Gordon GS, Cocks DL. Hospital drug formularies and use of hospital services. *Med Care.* 1993:31:851-867.

32. Morreim EH. Gaming the system: dodging the rules, ruling the dodgers. *Arch Intern Med.* 1991; 151:443-447.

33. Greco PJ, Eisenberg JM. Changing physicians' practices. *N. Eng. J. Med.* 1993:329:1271-1273.

34. Lomas J, Anderson GM, Domnick-Pierre K, Vayda E, Enkin MW, Hannah WJ. Do practice guidelines guide practice? The effect of a consensus statement on the practice of physicians. *N. Engl. J. Med.* 1989;321:1306-1311.

35. Blustein J, Marmor TR. Cutting waste by making rules: promises, pitfalls, and realistic prospects. *Univ Pa Law Rev.* 1992;140:1543-1572.

36. Tunis SR, Hayward RSA, Wilson MC, et al. Internists' attitudes about clinical practice guidelines. *Ann Intern Med.* 1994;120:956-963.

37. Kassirer JP. The quality of care and the quality of measuring it. *N. Engl. J. Med.* 1993:329:1263-1265.

38. Stein JH, ed. *Internal Medicine.* 2nd ed. Boston, Mass: Little Brown & Co Inc; 1987.

39. Weingarten SR, Riedinger MS, Conner L, et al. Practice guidelines and reminders to reduce duration of hospital stay for patients with chest pain: an interventional trial. *Ann Intern Med.* 1994; 120:257-263.

40. Steill IG, McKnight D, Greenberg GH, et al. Implementation of the Ottawa ankle rules. *JAMA.* 1994; 271:827-832.

41. Welch HG, Bernat JL. Mogielnicki RP. Who's in charge here? maximizing patient benefit and professional authority by physician limit setting. *J Gen Intern Med.* 1994;9:450-454.

42. Welch HG. Should the health care forest be selectively thinned by physicians or clear-cut by payers? *Ann Intern Med.* 1991;115:223-226.

43. Hadorn DC, ed. *Basic Benefits and Clinical Guidelines.* Boulder, Colo: Westview Press; 1992.

44. Welch HG, Larson EB. Dealing with limited resources:the Oregon decision to curtail funding for organ transplantation. *N. Engl. J. Med.* 1988; 319:171-173.

45. Eddy DM. Screening for cervical cancer. *Ann Intern Med.* 1990;113:214-226.

46. Drummond MF, Heyse J, Cook J, McGuire A. Selection of end points in economic evaluations of coronary heart-disease interventions. *Med Decis Making.* 1993:13:184-190.

47. Singer PA, Tasch ES, Stocking C, Rubin S, Siegler M, Weichselbaum R. Sex or survival: tradeoffs between quality and quantity of life. *J Clin Oncol.* 1991;9:328-334.

48. Hadorn DC. Setting health care priorities in Oregon:cost-effectiveness meets the rule of rescue. *JAMA.* 1991:265:2218-2225.

49. Schelling TC. The life you save may be your own. In: Chase SB, ed. *Problems in Public Expenditure Analysis.* Washington, DC: Brookings Institution: 1968.

50. Gore A. *Earth in the Balance: Ecology and the Human Spirit.* New York, NY: Plume Books: 1992.

CHAPTER 16

ETHICAL ISSUES IN MANAGED CARE

*Council on Ethical and Judicial Affairs,
American Medical Association*

*Members of the Council
on Ethical and Judicial Af-
fairs at the time of this re-
port include the following:
John Glasson, MD, Dur-
ham, NC, (Chair); Charles
W. Plows, MD, Anaheim,
Calif, (Vice Chair); Oscar
W. Clarke, MD, Gallipolis,
Ohio; Victoria Ruff, MD,
Columbus, Ohio; Drew
Fuller, Gainesville, Fla;
Craig H. Kliger, MD, Los
Angeles, Calif; George T.
Wilkins, Jr, MD, Ed-
wardsville, Ill; James H.
Cosgriff, Jr, MD, Buffalo,
NY Robert M. Tenery, Jr,
MD, Dallas, Tex; Kirk B.
Johnson, JD, Chicago, Ill
(Senior Vice President
and General Counsel and
Staff Author);David Orent-
licher, MD, JD, Chicago,
Ill (Secretary and Staff
Author); Karey M. Har-
wood, Somerville, Mass
(Staff Associate); Jeff
Leslie, New Haven, Conn
(Staff Associate and Staff
Author).*

A PRIMARY CONCERN OF MEDICAL ETHICISTS FOR SOME TIME HAS BEEN THE absence of any meaningful analysis of the impact of health care delivery marketplace changes and current legislative reforms on the essential tenets of the physician-patient relationship. Although President Clinton's original reform proposal addressed in broad terms the ethical imperatives supporting universal access, it left virtually unexamined the more fundamental question of the role of the physician in a reformed system in which the incentives are dramatically changed and budgets determine the amount of health care spending and services.

In June 1990, the Council issued a report, "Financial Incentives to Limit Care: Financial Implications for HMOs and IPAs,"[1] which described the financial incentives that managed care plans offer physicians to limit their provision of care. The report concluded that patient welfare must remain the first concern of physicians working in health maintenance organizations (HMOs) and independent practice associations (IPAs), and that physicians must disclose all relevant financial inducements and contractual restrictions that affect the delivery of health care to patients.

With its emphasis on managed care and managed competition, health system reform will greatly increase the salience of the ethical concerns raised by managed care. It is therefore essential that the profession and society act now to ensure that managed care techniques are implemented in a way that protects patients and the integrity of the patient-physician relationship.

In this report, the Council reiterates the physician's commitment to patient welfare first, and updates its previous recommendations for physicians. This report discusses in greater detail the potential conflicts of interest faced by physicians practicing in the managed care environment. It then recommends measures to preserve the fundamental duty of physicians as patient advocates by reducing the risk of rationing and inappropriate financial incentives.

BACKGROUND

As health care costs have risen and calls for more cost-conscious health care have been made,[2] health care insurers increasingly have adopted principles of managed care.[3] Several different types of managed care arrangements have managed care.[3] Several different types of managed care arrangements have gained prominence in the American health care system, including group- and staff-model HMOs, IPAs, and preferred provider organizations. Fee-for-service plans are also using many of the cost-saving techniques of managed care.

Managed care plans use a number of techniques. Some of them are directed at physician behavior. Others are directed at subscribers to the plan.[4,5] For example, managed care plans typically encourage subscribers to seek health care when it is still possible to prevent the development of illness by covering a broad range of preventive and primary care services. In addition, they restrict subscribers to panels of physicians who have agreed to accept lower reimbursements or who may have exhibited a history of practicing lower-cost care. Managed care plans can also control their subscribers' behavior by denying access to the services of medical specialists until the subscriber has obtained the approval of a primary care physician.

Managed care plans constrain the costs of participating physician practices in several ways as well. The plans may restrict the ability of physicians to perform certain procedures or to order certain medications or diagnostic tests. For example, a physician may need the approval of a radiologist before ordering a diagnostic imaging test, or a managed care plan might exclude some expensive drugs from the plan's formulary. Managed care plans aggressively use programs of utilization review to detect what they consider medically inappropriate or unnecessarily costly practice patterns.

Managed care plans can also reduce costs by creating economies of scale, by coordinating care among physicians and hospitals, by mandating the use of guidelines or parameters of care *(Chicago Tribune.* November 10, 1993:Al), and by establishing advanced information systems that provide an improved basis on which to measure quality and efficiency.

Managed care plans also encourage physicians to make cost-conscious treatment decisions through the use of financial incentives. The plans often compensate physicians with capitation fees or a salary. In addition, plans typically use incentives for physicians to limit their use of diagnostic tests, referrals to other physicians, hospital care, or other ancillary services. For example, managed care plans often pay bonuses to physicians, with the amount of the bonus increasing as the plans' expenditures for patient care decrease. Or plans often withhold a fixed percentage of their physicians' compensation until the end of the year to cover any shortfalls in the funds budgeted for expenditures on patient care. If there is no shortfall, or the shortfall can be covered by part of the withheld fees, the remaining withheld fees are returned to the physicians.[1]

While efforts to contain costs are critical, and while many of the approaches of managed care have an impact, managed care can compromise the quality and integrity of the patient-physician relationship and reduce the quality of care received by patients. In particular, by creating conflicting loyalties for the physician, some of the techniques of managed care can undermine the physician's fundamental obligation to serve as patient advocate.

Moreover, in their zeal to control utilization, managed care plans may withhold appropriate diagnostic procedures or treatment modalities for patients. Indeed, the US Department of Health and Human Services recently expressed concerns about practices at a major HMO after receiving eight allegations of insufficient patient care (*Wall Street Journal*, October 3, 1994:Al).

THE PATIENT-PHYSICIAN RELATIONSHIP

Before discussing the potential impact of managed care on the patient-physician relationship, it is important to consider what is at stake. The foundation of the patient-physician relationship is the trust that physicians are dedicated first and foremost to serving the needs of their patients. In the oath of Hippocrates, trust is a central element in almost all the ethical obligations of physicians: physicians must keep patients' private information confidential, avoid mischief and sexual misconduct, and give no harmful or death-causing agent. Patients can expect that physicians will come to their aid, even if it means putting the physician's own health at risk,[6] and they can trust that physicians will do everything in their power to help their patients. It is this trust that enables patients to communicate private information and to place their health, and indeed their lives, in the hands of their physicians.[1] Without trust, the success of the healing process would be seriously diminished.

No other party in the health care system has the kind of responsibility that physicians have to advocate for patients, and no other party is in a position to assume that kind of responsibility. Physicians care for patients directly, are in the best position to know patients' interests, and can advocate within the health care system for patients' needs. Without the commitment that physicians place patients' interests first, and act as agents for their patients alone, there is no assurance that the patient's health and well-being will be protected.

ETHICAL CONCERNS

Managed care involves at least two conflicting loyalties for the physician, conflicts that are not unique to managed care. First, physicians are expected to balance the interests of their patients with the interests of other patients. When deciding whether to order a test or procedure for a patient, the physician must consider whether the slot should be saved for another patient, or not used at all to conserve the plan's resources. Second, managed care can place the needs of patients in conflict with the financial interests of their physicians. Managed care plans use bonuses and fee withholdings to make physicians cost-conscious. As a result, when physicians are deciding whether to order a test, they will recognize that it may have an adverse impact on their income.

Some commentators argue that market forces will ensure that patients are protected from undue conflicts of interest. Because subscribers are theoretically free to choose their managed care organization based on quality of coverage, performance record and other factors, they can theoretically drive those managed care organizations with the least impressive records out of business. However, it is unlikely that these consumer choices alone will ensure high-quality managed care organizations. As stated in a recent editorial, "patient satisfaction depends more on visible amenities and personal relations than on the quality and appropriateness of medical services. . . ."[7]

The following two sections address the potential conflicts of interest for physicians under managed care.

Conflicts Among Patients

While some cost containment can be achieved by eliminating waste and inefficiency, it is also being achieved by limiting the availability of tests or procedures that offer only small or uncertain benefits, or that provide a likely benefit but at a great expense. Because managed care plans generally work within a limited budget and, increasingly, are for-profit companies that compete to report favorable results to shareholders,[7,8] the cost of a service will influence whether the service is offered to patients who might benefit from it. Allocation rules are developed by the plans to deal with this issue.

Managed care plans can make these allocation decisions in a number of ways: by developing guidelines that determine for a physician when the service should be offered, by instructing physicians to provide medically necessary care and delegating to the physicians the allocation decisions, or by some combination of allocation guidelines, physician discretion and oversight.

An example of an allocation decision might involve the use of high-osmolar contrast media (HOCM) and low-osmolar contrast media (LOCM) in diagnostic imaging procedures.[9] Both HOCM and LOCM produce images of similar quality and are approved by the Food and Drug Administration as safe and effective. Adverse reactions, including "changes in cardiac performance, alterations in renal function, depression of the central nervous system, pain at the site of injection, flushing, nausea, and vomiting,"[9] are somewhat more likely with the use of HOCM. In addition, fatal adverse reactions with both media are extremely rare and no more likely with HOCM than LOCM.[10(p616),11] However, there is a significant difference in the cost of the two media: LOCM are considerably more expensive than HOCM. Whereas a peripheral arteriography procedure would use about $10 worth of HOCM, the same procedure would use about $180 worth of LOCM, an increase of 18 times the HOCM cost.[9]

It is not obvious which contrast medium should be used. In fact, the decision to use HOCM or LOCM is essentially a value judgment about the relative costs and benefits of the two different media. While medical expertise is necessary to determine what benefits and risks are associated with the two media, the weighing of those benefits and risks with financial costs is not simply a medical decision but also a social judgment about the value of spending additional resources to lower health risks in this manner. A more difficult allocation case involves the use of bone marrow transplants for certain kinds of advanced cancer. The stakes for the patient are high – a prolonged life, if successful – but the costs are great and the likelihood of success uncertain. Some plans will restrict or discourage the treatment; others may make it available under some circumstances.[12]

Ethical Problems with Bedside Rationing. Physicians make cost benefit judgments every day as a part of their professional responsibility in treating patients. It is unethical to knowingly provide unnecessary care or to be wasteful in providing needed care.

Allocation judgments about costs and services that approach a "rationing" decision – the denial of a procedure that benefits a patient – are not part of the physician's traditional role and, indeed, conflict with it. Although physicians have traditionally served as de facto gatekeepers to the health care system, overseeing the public's use of medical care, the cost-primacy environment of managed care significantly complicates this role.[13] As Pellegrino has written, "This [gatekeeper] role is morally dubious because it generates a conflict between the responsibilities of the physician as a primary advocate of the patient and as guardian of society's resources."[13] While this responsibility to guard society's resources is an important one, physicians must remain primarily dedicated to the health care needs of their individual patients.

The primary care physician's role in managed care illustrates the ethical problems associated with bedside rationing. The physician-gatekeeper determines whether the patient will be granted further access to the health care system, including referrals to specialists and diagnostic tests. At the same time, the physician is required by rules and encouraged by incentives to be aware of the overall financial limitations of the managed care entity for which he or she works.[4] The physician knows that there are other patients who have subscribed to the managed care plan and who are owed a certain level of health care.[14] These competing concerns mean that a patient's further treatment depends not only on the physician's judgment about the legitimacy of that patient's present medical need but also on the relative weight of that need in comparison with the organization's need to serve all patients and control costs. Inconsistent and uninformed decisions are inevitable.

The primary care physician has the greatest responsibility within the managed care organization to assess the seriousness of patients' conditions accurately. A keen understanding of common and uncommon health problems is therefore required, as it is of all primary care physicians. However, the pressures of cost containment may encourage some physicians to try to manage cases longer than they should. Physicians may feel compelled to stretch their competence to keep patients at the primary care level and conserve resources. Inappropriate treatment and improper or missed diagnoses are potential outcomes of such decisions to delay or deny referral.

Preserving the Physician's Role. The physician is obligated to provide or recommend treatment when the physician believes that the treatment will materially benefit the patient, and not to withhold the treatment to preserve the plan's resources. Physicians should not engage in bedside rationing.

But many allocation decisions are within arguable ranges or gray areas of at least minimally acceptable treatment. There are two steps to reducing physician-patient conflict in these circumstances. First, allocation decisions should be determined not by individual physicians at the bedside but according to guidelines established at a higher policymaking level. Physicians should contribute their expertise in the development of the guidelines and should advocate for the consideration of differences among patients. For example, it might be advisable for a certain group of patients at high risk to be offered LOCM, while others who are not in this group are offered HOCM. Physicians can help ensure that all medically relevant information is considered, and that no group of patients is put at an unfair disadvantage.

Second, and more importantly, even if the use of the LOCM were prohibited by a guideline for all or a particular class of patients, it remains the physician's duty to recommend its use and to advocate for the patient's right to the treatment in any case in which material benefit to a particular patient would result.

The structure through which physicians offer their expertise in policy-level decisions is very important. To help define this structure, the American Medical Association (AMA) recently proposed legislation[15] that would require managed care organizations to establish a medical staff structure, much like that in existence in every hospital in the United States. The proposal includes a governing board for the managed care organization that would include at least three physician members as representatives of participating physicians, and a medical board composed entirely of participating physicians. Physicians on the medical board would be responsible for periodically reviewing restrictions on services to subscribers and other issues related to health care coverage. They would also review quality of care and physician credentialing on a periodic basis and disclose their review criteria to subscribers. The governing board would be ultimately responsible for the activities of the managed care organization, but participating physicians would have formal mechanisms for input and responsibilities on crucial medical practice issues.

In addition to the physician's role in making rationing decisions, there is an equally critical role for patients. The decision-making process should include some mechanism for taking into account the preferences and values of the people whom the rationing decision will most directly affect.[14] Accurate and full disclosure is most important. In addition, a managed care organization could use "town meetings" and other mechanisms whereby subscribers could voice their preferences or "vote" on what treatments should be included in their benefits package.

Once guidelines and criteria are developed at the policy level, physicians' are free to make clinical decisions based on those guidelines and criteria. For example, if a managed care plan decided to offer LOCM only to patients at high risk for an adverse reaction to HOCM, physicians would decide which patients are at high risk.

In addition to the development of appropriate procedures for making allocation decisions, there are other steps that must be taken to protect patient welfare when the allocation procedures are implemented. For example, as part of the process of giving patients informed consent to treatment, physicians should disclose all available treatment alternatives, regardless of cost, including those potentially beneficial treatments that are not offered under the terms of the plan. As described in the Council's report on financial incentives to limit care,[1] obligations of disclosure always apply to the physician practicing in managed care. With full understanding of the limitations affecting their treatment, patients will have the opportunity to make alternative arrangements for care that is not available in their health plan. Thus, for example, if the health plan did not cover a particular pharmaceutical that the physician might otherwise have prescribed, the patient could choose to pay out-of-pocket for the pharmaceutical.

It is also critical for managed care plans to have a well-structured appeals process through which physicians and patients can challenge the denial of a particular diagnostic test or therapeutic procedure. Such a process should afford the physician an opportunity to advocate on the patient's behalf before the plan's medical board or governing board. Appeals mechanisms for treatment denials are essential because policy-level allocation decisions can never fully account for all contingencies and will sometimes underserve individual patients. Managed care plans, as institutions, have an ethical responsibility to allow patients to challenge treatment decisions that directly affect their health and well-being.

In some circumstances, physicians have an obligation to initiate appeals on behalf of their patients. Cases may arise in which a health plan has an allocation guideline that is generally fair, but in particular circumstances results in unfair denials of care, i.e., denial of care that would materially benefit the patient. In such cases, the physician's duty as patient advocate requires that the physician challenge the denial and argue for the provision of treatment in the specific case. Cases may also arise in which a health plan has an allocation guideline that is generally unfair in its operation. In such cases, the physician's duty as patient advocate requires not only a challenge to any denials of treatment from the guideline but also advocacy at the health plan's policymaking level to seek an elimination or modification of the guideline.

Conflicts Between Physician and Patient

Ethical Problems With Financial Incentives to Limit Care. As discussed herein, managed care plans encourage physicians to be more cost-conscious by using bonuses, fee withholds, and other financial incentives to limit care. With these incentives, physicians recognize that they may reduce their income when they order tests, hospitalize patients, or provide other services. The incentives are not inherently unethical, but they can be depending on their design and intensity.

There are two important ways in which financial incentives to limit care compromise the physician's duty of loyalty to patient care. First, physicians have an incentive to cut corners in their patient care, by temporizing too long, eschewing extra diagnostic tests, or refraining from an expensive referral. Several studies have tried to measure the health outcomes of patients in managed care or prepaid settings against the health outcomes of patients in fee-for-service arrangements. Although disturbing anecdotes abound, these studies have found largely mixed results:[16] harm or inadequate health outcomes have not been conclusively demonstrated in managed care arrangements,[17-18] although these patients may be at an increased risk of harm.[19-21] Second, even in the absence of actual patient harm, the incentives may erode patient trust as patients wonder whether they are receiving all necessary care or are being denied care because of the physicians' pecuniary concerns.

Physicians must place patients' interests ahead of their own interests, including financial remuneration.[1] Financial conflicts are inherent in the practice of medicine, regardless of the system of delivery, and physicians generally have been able to maintain their duty to patient welfare despite those conflicts. However, incentives to limit care are more problematic than incentives to provide care.

First, financial incentives to limit care exploit the financial motive of physicians, making the physician's financial self-interest indispensable for the success of the managed care organization. Second, financial incentives to limit care are less likely than financial incentives created by fee-for-service to coincide with patients' interests, because patients generally prefer the risk of too much care to the risk of too little care. Third, the effects of incentives to limit care are less likely to be noticed by patients. When a physician recommends a course of action under fee-for-service reimbursement, the patient can seek a second opinion. However, when a physician does not offer an intervention under managed care, the patient may have no idea that a treatment option was withheld, and therefore not recognize the need for a second opinion.[8]

Not all financial incentives to limit care create the same conflict of interest between the physician's and patient's interests. In general, the greater the strength of the incentive, the more likely it will create a serious conflict of interest that could lead to patient harm. The strength of a financial incentive to limit care can be judged by various factors, including the percentage of the physician's income placed at risk, the frequency with which incentive payments are calculated, and the size of the group of physicians on which the economic performance is judged.[22]

If the managed care plan places 20% of a physician's income at risk, the physician likely will be much more conscious of costs than if the plan places 5% of income at risk. Similarly, if a physician's incentive payments are based solely on his or her treatment decisions, there is a strong incentive to limit services for each patient. When payments are based on the performance of a group of physicians, on the other hand, the incentive is diminished. When physicians are placed at risk together, they have an incentive to ensure that their colleagues are practicing in a cost-effective manner, and the incentive payments will be based on costs incurred by a large patient pool. When the patient panel is small, there is a risk that treatment costs will be skewed by an unrepresentative group of patients that have unusually high-cost needs for medical care.

The strength of a financial incentive can also vary with the frequency of incentive payments. If payments are made on a monthly basis rather than a yearly basis, the physician receives rapid feedback on the economic consequences of treatment decisions, and is therefore likely to be more sensitive to those consequences. In addition, when incentives are calculated on a monthly basis, there is less of an opportunity for the costs of cases that are above-average to be offset by the costs of cases that are below-average. Accordingly there is a stronger incentive not to incur unusually high expenses in any one case. Because of this concern, the Health Care Financing Administration, in its proposed rules, would permit managed care plans to place less of their physicians' income at risk if the plans calculate their incentive payments more frequently than once a year.[23]

Preserving the Physician's Role. Before the Council discusses its recommendations for dealing with financial incentives to limit care, it is important to mention that the AMA is precluded from issuing restrictive guidelines in this area. A Federal Trade Commission order that was upheld by the US Supreme Court prohibits the AMA from "regulating" or "advising on the ethical propriety of . . . the consideration offered or provided to any physician in any contract with any entity that offers physicians' services to the public."[24]

The most effective way to eliminate inappropriate conflicts is to create the use of financial incentives based on quality rather than quantity of services. Reimbursement that serves to promote a standard of "appropriate" behavior helps to maintain the goals of professionalism. Unlike incentives based on quantity of services, which punish the provision of both appropriate and inappropriate services, incentives based on quality of care punish only inappropriate services.

Judgments about the quality of a physician's practice should reflect several measures. First, it is essential to consider objective outcomes data, including data about mortality and morbidity, corrected for caseload. Second, because outcomes are often beyond the physician's control, it is important to consider the degree to which the physician adheres to practice guidelines or other standards of care. Third, patient satisfaction should be considered. Although patients are limited in their ability to evaluate physician competence, they are the best judges of one critical quality of physician care, the physician's bedside manner. In addition, patient satisfaction reflects the extent to which the physician has accommodated the goals of the patient as required by the patient's right to exercise self-determination in medical care. Fourth, the judgments of a physician's peers should be considered; these judgments provide an important assessment of quality that may be particularly useful "in areas that are difficult to assess reliably with other measures."[25(p1658)]

Because measurements of quality are still in the rudimentary stages of development, it is important to ensure that other safeguards are in place to prevent abuse from incentives based on quantity of care. Reasonable limits should be placed on the extent to which a physician's ordering of services can affect his other income. For example, quantitative financial incentives should be calculated on groups of physicians rather than individual physicians.

PATIENT AUTONOMY AND RESPONSIBILITY

Many commentators argue that managed care threatens patient autonomy because it curtails patients' freedom of choice. Patients are usually limited in their choice of primary care physicians and, to a much greater degree, specialists, and they are sometimes limited in their choice of treatments. Patients may not be able to receive a desired diagnostic test or referral, and their freedom to personally tailor treatment can be thwarted. In addition, continuity of care may be disrupted if a patient is forced, for a variety of reasons, to change physicians to keep their health care benefits.[26]

Public participation in the formulation of benefits packages may resolve some of these concerns about limited autonomy. Legislation reasonably protecting patients' rights to be informed and to choose, and protecting physicians' rights to remain professionals is also essential. Patients can exercise their autonomy by participating in the decisions of their health plan or in government processes that may restrict their choices or benefits. In addition, patients have a responsibility to learn as much as they can about their choices of plans, including the exact nature of the different benefits packages and their limitations. Patients have a responsibility to make sure they know and understand the terms of their own health care plan.

As patient advocates, physicians continue to have duties of disclosure. They must ensure that all treatment alternatives, regardless of cost, are disclosed. They must also ensure that the managed care organization has fulfilled its obligation to disclose the terms of the benefits package, including all limitations and restrictions.

Patient autonomy does not guarantee the right to have all treatment choices funded. Some limits on personal freedom are inevitable in a society that tries to provide all of its members with adequate health care. The desire for accurate diagnosis and use of technological medical care, no matter how little the benefit, has been cited as a major factor in increasing health care costs in this country.[27] Moreover, patient autonomy entails patient responsibility, including a responsibility to abide by societal decisions to conserve health care and to make an individual effort to use resources wisely and lead a healthy lifestyle.

While physicians must remain patient advocates, patients do not have an unlimited claim to physicians' obligation to provide health care. Physicians should not manipulate or "game" the system to answer patients' demands.[28]

To fully exercise their autonomy, patients need to be fully informed about the philosophy and goals of managed care. In an earlier report, the Council stated that the physician's responsibilities under managed care include a duty to disclose to the patient conflicts of interest that may affect patient care and medical alternatives that cannot be offered because of the restrictions of the managed care plan. That report specifically states that physicians have a duty to disclose financial incentives, to disclose contractual agreements restricting referral, and to ensure that the managed care plan makes adequate disclosure of the details of the plan to subscribers.[1,29]

GUIDELINES

For the reasons described in this report, the Council on Ethical and Judicial Affairs issues the following guidelines:

1. The duty of patient advocacy is a fundamental element of the physician-patient relationship that should not be altered by the system of health care delivery in which physicians practice. Physicians must continue to place the interests of their patients first.

2. When managed care plans place restrictions on the care that physicians in the plan may provide to their patients, the following principles should be followed:

   (a) Any broad allocation guidelines that restrict care and choices – which go beyond the cost-benefit judgments made by physicians as a part of their normal professional responsibilities – should be established at a policymaking level so that individual physicians are not asked to engage in ad hoc bedside rationing.

   (b) Regardless of any allocation guidelines or gatekeeper directives, physicians must advocate for any care they believe will materially benefit their patients.

   (c) Physicians should be given an active role in contributing their expertise to any allocation process and should advocate for guidelines that are sensitive to differences among patients. Managed care plans should create structures similar to hospital medical staffs that allow physicians to have meaningful input into the plan's development of allocation guidelines. Guidelines for allocating health care should be reviewed on a regular basis and updated to reflect advances in medical knowledge and changes in relative costs.

   (d) Adequate appellate mechanisms for both patients and physicians should be in place to address disputes regarding medically necessary care. In some circumstances, physicians have an obligation to initiate appeals on behalf of their patients. Cases may arise in which a health plan has an allocation guideline that is generally fair, but in particular circumstances results in unfair denials of care that, in the physician's judgment, would materially benefit the patient. In such cases, the physician's duty as patient advocate requires that the physician challenge the denial and argue for the provision of treatment in the specific case. Cases may also arise in which a health plan has an allocation guideline that is generally unfair in its operation. In such cases, the physician's duty as patient advocate requires not only a challenge to any denials of treatment from the guideline but also advocacy at the health plan's policymaking level to seek an elimination or modification of the guideline. Physicians should assist patients who wish to seek additional appropriate care outside the plan when the physician believes the care is in the patient's best interests.

   (e) Managed care plans must adhere to the requirement of informed consent that patients be given full disclosure of material information. Full disclosure requires that managed care plans inform potential subscribers of limitations or restrictions on the benefits package when they are considering entering the plan.

   (f) Physicians also should continue to promote full disclosure to patients enrolled in managed care organizations. The physician's obligation to disclose treatment alternatives to patients is not altered by any limitations in the coverage provided by the patient's managed care plan. Full disclosure includes informing patients of all their treatment options, even those that may not be covered under the terms of the managed care plan. Patients may then determine whether an appeal is appropriate or whether they wish to seek care outside the plan for treatment alternatives that are not covered.

(g) Physicians should not participate in any plan that encourages or requires care at or below minimum professional standards.

3. When physicians are employed or reimbursed by managed care plans that offer financial incentives to limit care, serious potential conflicts are created between the physicians' personal financial interests and the needs of their patients. Efforts to contain health care costs should not place patient welfare at risk. Thus, financial incentives are permissible only if they promote the cost-effective delivery of health care and not the withholding of medically necessary care.

(a) Any incentives to limit care must be disclosed fully to patients by plan administrators on enrollment and at least annually thereafter.

(b) Limits should be placed on the magnitude of fee withholds, bonuses, and other financial incentives to limit care. Calculating incentive payments according to the performance of a sizable group of physicians rather than on an individual basis should be encouraged.

(c) Health plans or other groups should develop financial incentives based on quality of care. Such incentives should complement financial incentives based on the quantity of services used.

4. Patients have an individual responsibility to be aware of the benefits and limitations of their health care coverage. Patients should exercise their autonomy by public participation in the formulation of benefits packages and by prudent selection of health care coverage that best suits their needs.

KEY IDEAS FROM THIS ARTICLE:

- The foundation of the patient-physician relationship is the trust that physicians are dedicated first and foremost to serving the needs of their patients.

- Without the commitment that physicians place patients' interests first and act as agents for their patients alone, there is no assurance that the patient's health and well-being will be protected.

- By creating conflicting loyalties for the physician, some of the techniques of managed care can undermine the physician's fundamental obligation to serve as patient advocate.

- One conflicitng loyalty is that physicians are expected to balance the interests of their patients with the interests of other patients.

- A second conflicting loyalty is that managed care can place the needs of patients in conflict with the financial interests of their physicians.

- The duty of patient advocacy is a fundamental element of the physician-patient relationship that should not be altered by the system of health care delivery in which physicians practice.

- Any broad allocation guidelines should be established at a policymaking level so that individual physicians are not asked to engage in ad hoc bedside rationing.

- Physicians must advocate for any care they believe will materially benefit their patients.

- Physicians should be given an active role in contributing their expertise to any allocation process.

- Adequate appellate mechanisms for both patients and physicians should be in place to address disputes regarding medically necessary care.

- Physicians should promote full disclosure, which includes informing patients of all their treatment options, even those that may not be covered under the terms of the managed care plan.

- Patients have a responsibility to be aware of the limits and benefits of their coverage, to participate in the formulation of benefits packages, and to prudently select coverage that best suits their needs.

A SUGGESTED PROCESS FOR REFLECTING ON THIS ARTICLE:

(see pages 234-254 for other processes that might better fit your specific goals and objectives).

Not seldom, the words we use are ambiguous. Each person can have a different, sometimes opposite understanding of the words used to discuss an issue. Good ethics requires that the key concepts of a discussion be clarified and examined to uncover such divergent meanings and to develop consensual meaning.

Issue:	Key term(s) in this issue:	These term(s) mean to me:
1. Without the commitment that physicians place patients' interests first and act as agents for their patients alone, there is no assurance that the patient's health and well-being will be protected.		
2. One conflicting loyalty is that physicians are expected to balance the interests of their patients with the interests of other patients.		
3. The duty of patient advocacy is a fundamental element of the physician-patient relationship that should not be altered by the system of health care delivery in which physicians practice.		

Issue:	Key term(s) in this issue:	These term(s) mean to me:
4. Physicians must advocate for any care they believe will materially benefit their patients.		
5. Adequate appellate mechanisms for both patients and physicians should be in place to address disputes regarding medically necessary care.		

IN LIGHT OF OUR DISCUSSION:

• as (executive committee, ethics committee, etc.), what are some next steps that we should take?

• as (hospital, home health agency, etc.), what are some next steps that we should take?

• what systems and structures call for special attention in order to improve the situation?

ENDNOTES

1. Council on Ethical and Judicial Affairs, American Medical Association. Financial incentives to limit care: financial implications for HMOs and IPAs. In: *Code of Medical Ethics: Reports of the Council on Ethical and Judicial Affairs of the American Medical Association, Vol. I,* Chicago, Ill: American Medical Association; 1990:130-135.

2. Enthoven A, Kronick R. A consumer-choice health plan for the 1990s: universal health insurance in a system designed to promote quality and economy. *N. Engl. J. Med.* 1989;320:29-37.

3. Povar G, Moreno J. Hippocrates and the health maintenance organization. *Ann Intern Med.* 1988; 109:419-424.

4. Iglehart JK. The American health care system: managed care. *N. Engl. J. Med.* 1992;327:742-747.

5. American Medical Association. *Principles of Managed Care: A Summary of American Medical Association Policy.* Chicago, Ill: American Medical Association; 1993.

6. Council on Ethical and Judicial Affairs, American Medical Association. Ethical issues involved in the growing AIDS crisis. *JAMA* 1988;259:1360-1361.

7. Relman AS. Medical practice under the Clinton reforms. *N. Engl. J. Med.* 1993;329:1574-1576.

8. Lorreim EH. Cost containment: challenging fidelity and justice. *Hastings Cent Rep.* 1988;18(6): 20-25.

9. American Medical Association. How cost containment may affect the standard of care in medical malpractice litigation. In: *Proceedings of the House of Delegates of the American Medical Association: 140th Annual Meeting.* Chicago, Ill: American Medical Association: 1991:121-136.

10. Bettman MA. Ionic versus nonionic contrast agents for intravenous use: are all the answers in? *Radiology.* 1990;175:616-618.

11. Katayama H, Yamaguchi K, Kozuka T, Takashima T, Seez P, Matsuura K. Adverse reactions to ionic and nonionic contrast media: a report from the Japanese Committee on the Safety of Contrast Media. *Radiology.* 1990;175:621-628.

12. Peters WP, Rogers M. Variation in approval by insurance companies of coverage for autologous bone marrow transplantation for breast cancer. *N. Engl. J. Med.* 1994;330:473-477.

13. Pellegrino ED. Rationing health care: the ethics of medical gatekeeping. *J Contemp Health Law Policy.* 1986;2:3-45.

14. Council on Ethical and Judicial Affairs. American Medical Association. Ethical issues in health care system reform: the provision of adequate health care. *JAMA.* 1994;272:1056-1062.

15. American Medical Association. *Physician Health Plans and Networks Act of 1994.* Chicago. Ill: American Medical Association; 1994.

16. Miller RH, Luft HS. Managed care plan performance since 1980: a literature analysis. *JAMA.* 1994;271:1512-1519.

17. Rubenstein LV, Kahn KL, Reinisch E, et al. Changes in quality of care for five diseases measured by implicit review, 1981 to 1986. *JAMA* 1990; 264:1974-1979.

18. Kahn KL, Keeler EB, Sherwood MJ, et al. Comparing outcomes of care before and after implementation of the DRG-based prospective payment system. *JAMA.* 1990:264:1984-1988.

19. Kosecoff J, Kahn KL, Rogers WH. et al. Prospective payment system and impairment at discharge: the 'quicker-and-sicker' story revisited *JAMA.* 1990:264:1980-19.

20. Ware JE Jr, Brook RH, Rogers WH, et al. Comparison of health outcomes at a health maintenance organization with those of fee-for-service. *Lancet.* 1986;1:1017-1022.

21. Clement DG, Retchin SM, Brown RS, Stegall MH. Access and outcomes of elderly patients enrolling in managed care. *JAMA* 1994;271:1487-1492.

22. US General Accounting Office. *Medicare: Physicians Incentive Payments by Prepaid Health Plans Could Lower Quality of Care.* Washington, DC: US Government Printing Office: 1988:23-27.

23. Health Care Financing Administration, US Dept. of Health and Human Services. Medicare and Medicaid programs: requirements for physician incentive plans in prepaid health care organizations. *Federal Register.* 1992;57:59024-59040.

24. Federal Trade Commission Order. Docket No. 9064. *JAMA.* 1982;248:981-982.

25. Ramsey PG, Wenrich, MD, Carline JD, Inui TS, Larson EB, JP. Use of peer ratings to evaluate physician performance. *JAMA.* 1993:269:1655-1660.

26. Emanuel EJ, Brett AS. Managed competition and the patient-physician relationship. *N. Engl. J. Med.* 1993;329:879-882.

27. Kassirer JP. Our stubborn quest for diagnostic certainty: a cause of excessive testing. *N Engl J.* Fred. 1989:320:1489-1491.

28. Morreim EH. Gaming the system: dodging the rules, ruling the dodgers. *Arch Intern Med.* 1991; 151:443-447.

29. Council on Ethical and Judicial Affairs, American Medical Association. Opinion 8.13: referral of patient – disclosure of limitations. In: *Code of Medical Ethics: Current Opinions With Annotations.* Chicago, Ill: American Medical Association; 1994.

CHAPTER 17

PRESERVING THE PHYSICIAN-PATIENT RELATIONSHIP IN THE ERA OF MANAGED CARE

Ezekiel J. Emanuel, MD, PhD, Nancy Neveloff Dubler, LLB

EVEN WITHOUT COMPREHENSIVE HEALTH CARE REFORM LEGISLATION, the US health care system is undergoing significant changes. Probably the most important change is the expansion of managed care with significant price competition. One of the major concerns about this change is the effect of managed care on the physician-patient relationship. To provide a normative standard for evaluating the effect of changes, we need an ideal conception of the physician-patient relationship. This ideal can be summarized by six C's: choice, competence, communication, compassion, continuity, and (no) conflict of interest. For the 37 million uninsured Americans, there is little chance of realizing the ideal physician-patient relationship, since they lack the choice of practice setting and physician, receive care in a rushed atmosphere that undermines communication and compassion, and have no continuity of care. While many insured Americans may believe they have an ideal physician-patient relationship, the relationship is threatened by lack of a regular assessment of competence, by financial incentives that undermine good communication, and by the persistence of conflict of interest. The shift to managed care may: improve the choice of practice settings, especially in sections of the country that currently lack managed care; increase choice of preventive services; make quality assessments more routine; and improve communication by making greater use of primary care physicians and nonphysician providers, However, the expansion of managed care and the imposition of significant cost control have the potential to undermine all aspects of the ideal physician-patient relationship. Choice could be restricted by employers and by managed care selection of physicians; poor quality indicators could undermine assessments of competence; productivity requirements could eliminate time necessary for communication; changing from one to another managed care plan to secure the lowest costs could produce significant disruption in continuity of care; and use of salary schemes that reward physicians for not using medical services could increase conflict of interest.

— *JAMA*, 1995;273:323-329

Major health care system reform legislation died – or was killed – in the last Congress. Yet changes in our health care system are continuing, even accelerating. The most obvious change is the ever-expanding use of managed care, especially to control rising health care costs. The debate over managed care has tended to focus on whether – and how – it can control cost[1-3] No one doubts that this is a fundamental issue. Nevertheless, the tremendous changes brought about by the widespread implementation of managed care will extend beyond health care costs. While some have raised questions about the effect of managed care on use of technology and patient satisfaction, there has been woefully little discussion of other probable and important consequences, such as restrictions on local research, the probable reduced funding for physician training programs, and the closing of hospitals in rural areas and small communities.[4,5] In addition, little attention has been paid to how managed care might affect the physician-patient relationship. Yet, the public outcry over choice of physician in the recent debates about health care system reform has made clear that this is a major concern for the vast majority of citizens, whose interaction with the health care system is principally, if not exclusively, as patients. Thus, one of the fundamental questions for most Americans about the changes fostered by managed care is, How will managed care affect my relationship with my physician?

THE IDEAL PHYSICIAN-PATIENT RELATIONSHIP

To evaluate the effects of managed care, we need to delineate an ideal conception of the physician-patient relationship[6] This ideal establishes the normative standard for assessing the effect of the current health care system, as well as changes in the system. Although patients receive health care from a diverse number of providers, and the use of nonphysician providers, such as nurse practitioners, physician assistants, and nurse midwives, is likely to increase with more emphasis on primary care and managed care, we chose to concentrate on the physician-patient relationship. The reasons for this focus are many: physicians outnumber nonphysician providers; most Americans continue to receive their health care from physicians rather than nonphysician providers; there have been many more years, indeed, centuries, for reflection on the elements that constitute the ideal physician-patient relationship, while the ethical guidelines and legal rulings on nonphysician provider-patient relationships are more recent and have not been as exhaustively developed; and there is substantially more empirical research on the physician-patient relationship with which to formulate educated projections. Where relevant, we explore how relationships between physicians and nonphysician providers might affect interactions with patients. Americans have intuitions about what they consider to be ideal physician-patient relationship. These intuitions are personified in books, television programs, and other media through the portrayals of physicians, such as Marcus Welby. In addition, much has been written by physicians, ethicists, and lawyers about what constitutes the ideal physician-patient relationship.[7-19] In characterizing the many facets of the ideal physician-patient relationship, we try to specify and organize these intuitions, and then refine them by comparing them with the ideal explicitly defined in the literature and by the standards of practice embodied in ethical guidelines, legal rulings, and health care policies.[20-22] No characterization of this ideal will receive universal assent; physicians, ethicists and lawyers disagree among themselves about how to articulate the ideal physician-patient relationship. Often these disagreements are a result of emphasizing different aspects of the relationship rather than unbridgeable philosophical differences. Despite these differences, we believe it is possible to elucidate core understandings that are widely, if not uniformly, shared.

It is also important to recognize that this ideal evolves over time. Traits admired decades ago may no longer be revered, while other traits have become more prominent. For instance, paternalism might have been the accepted norm previously, but today respect for patient autonomy is widely agreed to be a core facet of the ideal physician-patient relationship. In addition, the ideal may not describe actual physician-patient relationships.[6,9] Physicians may not recognize or may fail to fulfill their duties, or adverse practice conditions may interfere with the realization of the ideal. Nevertheless, the fundamental elements of the ideal physician-patient relationship seem to be enduring and define the goal toward which we aspire. We measure our achievement by the ideal, even when we fall short.

We suggest that the fundamental elements of the ideal physician-patient relationship that are embodied in our intuitions and common to ethical analyses and legal standards can be expressed as six C's: choice, competence, communication, compassion, continuity, and (no) conflict of interest. While many people emphasize the importance of trust in the physician-patient relationship, we believe trust is the culmination of realizing these six C's, not an independent element.

Choice

As became clear in the debate over President Clinton's health care system reform proposal, many Americans consider choice to be a critical dimension of the ideal physician-patient relationship.[23-25] Four critical dimensions of this choice are (1) choice of practice type and setting, (2) choice of primary care physician, (3) choice of a specialist or special facility in an emergency or for a special condition, and (4) choice among treatment alternatives.[7,12,14,17,18] Patients want to be able to choose whether to receive their care from an independent practitioner or in an integrated health care system. More important, they also want to be able to choose who provides them with routine health care, to find a person with whom they have a rapport and to whom they can entrust their secrets and confidences. They fear being forced to receive care from a physician with whom they do not get along. If they confront a serious threat to their health, such as requiring major surgery or being diagnosed with cancer, patients want to be sure they can choose to go to "the best." For many Americans, choice of the best is a critical element in feeling that "no stone will be left unturned" when a major illness arises.[23,24] Finally, when there are several appropriate treatment options for a condition, such as mastectomy or breast-conserving therapy for breast cancer, Americans want to be able to choose for themselves which one to receive. This is the element of choice embodied in informed consent.[12,14,16-18] The tremendous emphasis Americans place on choice can sometimes appear as a fetish,[26,27] but we value it as one component of self-determination, a central ideal of American culture.[7,8,12,14-16,20,24]

Competence

Patients expect their physicians to be competent. While technical proficiency may not be sufficient, it is a necessary precondition for having a good physician-patient relationship; physicians who lack technical expertise cannot meet the ideal. Competence entails four elements. Physicians must possess (1) a good fund of knowledge that is kept current with developing practices; (2) good technical skills to perform diagnostic and therapeutic procedures; (3) good clinical judgment to differentiate important signs and symptoms from secondary ones, to know what diagnostic tests to utilize in what order, and to select the most appropriate therapies; and (4) an understanding of their own limitations and a willingness to consult specialists or other health care providers as required by the situation.[8,9,13,17,18]

Communication

An ideal physician-patient relationship requires good communication. First, good communication means that physicians listen to and understand the patient and communicate their understanding. This entails understanding the patient's symptoms, the patient's values, the effect of the disease on the patient's life, family, job and other pursuits, and any other health-related concerns the patient deems important.[7-14,16-19] In addition, patients should be able to tell their physicians what kind of information they want and do not want to know. For example, some patients with cancer prefer not to know their prognosis or a detailed delineation of the side-effects of treatment alternatives. In circumstances where patients, especially children and adolescents, may not be especially articulate or may be confronting new experiences that they have difficulty characterizing, physicians must be able to help patients explicate their experiences, values and feelings.[9-12,14,16,19]

Good communication skills also mean that physicians are capable of explaining to patients, in clear and comprehensible language, the nature of their disease, the diagnostic and therapeutic treatment alternatives available, and how these alternatives are likely to fulfill or undermine the patients' values. In this sense, physicians offer advice and direction that guide their patients through the issues raised by their illness and possible treatments.[7,9,10,12,14,16,17] For example, the physician can help patients with arthritis assess how alternative treatment options will help achieve their goals of functional independence and freedom from pain.

By strengthening the bond between patients and physicians, good communication prevents arguments, understandings and disputes. When communication is good, patients are less likely to misinterpret the information they receive, more willing to ask for clarification when information is unclear, quicker to call if symptoms fail to resolve. Good communication thus can mitigate the occurrence of negative events that lead to malpractice litigation.[31,32]

Compassion

Patients not only want technically proficient physicians, they also want empathic physicians.[33] Empathy from their physician enables patients to feel supported during times of great stress. This may be especially important for adolescents, whose health problems may also cause strains in their family. This is not to suggest that compassionate physicians simply reaffirms whatever values, feelings and experiences patients have.[9,10,16,19,23] Sometimes physicians see the need to help patients reconsider and revise their values, overcome their feelings, and place their experiences in a larger perspective. But these efforts are all undertaken with the intention of demonstrating compassion for the patient.[9,10,16,19,23]

Continuity

Once established, a patient's relationship with a competent and compassionate physician who is providing most of his or her care should endure over time.[7-10,12,13,16,17,19,24] The establishment of an ideal physician-patient relationship requires a significant investment of time. Patients frequently must search to identify a physician whom they consider competent and with whom they can communicate. It also takes time for physicians to understand and empathize with patients' values and feelings and to be able to help patients identify and utilize health care services that are appropriate for their condition and life situation.

Trusting relationships ensure that in times of stress, patients can rely on their physicians, secure in the knowledge that their history, attachments, values and feelings are understood. If patients are frequently forced to change physicians, it is hard for them to develop a deep and understanding relationship. An ongoing relationship is particularly important for patients who have chronic conditions such as arthritis, diabetes, or cancer and require repeated medical interventions over time. It may also be important for younger patients for whom choices by the patient or the patient's parents can profoundly affect future life prospects. Decisions to adopt healthy habits, to stop smoking to spare a child from passive smoke, or to bear painful but efficacious therapies are more likely to be made if recommended by a trusted physician in the context of an ongoing relationship.

Relationships that endure over time may be more efficient. Knowing a patient means that a physician more easily identifies therapies appropriate for the personality and capabilities of the patient. The physician will know what support services the patient can draw on. Similarly, patients are more likely to accept recommendations to "wait and see" or to delay expensive diagnostic testing from a physician in whom they have confidence, by virtue of having established a trusting relationship.

(No) Conflict of Interest

We expect that a physician's primary concern will be his or her patient's well-being, even though physicians may have obligations that conflict. Attending to the well-being of one patient may conflict with caring for another patient.[14] Sadly, it is well-recognized that caring for a patient may conflict with – and even be superseded by – the need to protect the interests of a third party.[7,12,14,17,35,36] Nevertheless, we do expect that the physician's care of a patient and concern for the patient's well-being will take precedence over the physician's own personal interests, especially financial interests.[7,12,13,15,17,18] This means that in a fee-for-service environment, physicians should not order procedures merely for their personal financial enrichment.[37] Conversely, in a capitated system, physicians should not withhold appropriate medical services to increase their own financial rewards. These expectations inform the rules restricting conflict of interest.[38-41]

THE PHYSICIAN-PATIENT RELATIONSHIP IN THE CURRENT HEALTH CARE SYSTEM

Uninsured Patients

At any one time, approximately 37 million Americans are uninsured, almost 25% of whom are children, and it is estimated that fully 63 million Americans go without insurance for at least one month during each 28-month period.[42] For these uninsured people without a regular physician, the current system precludes the possibility of having an ideal physician-patient relationship. Without health insurance or significant financial resources, the uninsured do not have any meaningful choice of health care setting or of a primary care physician.[43] They are often forced to forgo regular care or to receive their regular health care from emergency departments, public hospitals, or similar institutions that provide care to the uninsured.[23] Many physicians who work in these institutions are highly trained professionals, dedicated to serving the poor and to providing high-quality care to the uninsured. Yet in such settings, the uninsured will often see a different physician at each visit, in a rushed atmosphere where overworked staff tend to proceed at a frenzied pace. And the frequent changes in health insurance coverage, going from insured to uninsured and back to insured over a few years, disrupt continuity of care. Health care provided under these conditions precludes good communication or continuity. Even if the health care providers are individually competent, compassionate and dedicated, and have no financial conflicts of interest, it appears that uninsured patients do have worse health outcomes, which casts doubt on the competence of the total care they receive and highlights that outcomes depend on more than the qualities of health care providers.[44,45] While competence and compassion are essential elements of an ideal physician-patient relationship, they are insufficient without patient choice, good communication, and continuity. Thus, for millions of uninsured Americans, impersonal care has all but displaced caring and enduring physician-patient relationships.

Insured Patients

Many Americans with health insurance – or, rarely, with independent financial means – have been able to choose a physician they believe to be competent and caring and with whom they can communicate about their health care. More than two-thirds of Americans have maintained such a relationship over many years.[23,24] In some instances the physician has become as much a family friend as a provider of medical services. As the statistics on high patient satisfaction with their current physician demonstrate, many Americans believe their relationship with their physician is close to the ideal.[23,24] But even for them, some of the characteristics of the current system jeopardize that good relationship.

There are many ways in which choice of physician and choice of procedures are currently limited, even for insured Americans. Insurance companies and managed care plans may discourage utilization of or exclude coverage for certain physicians, procedures and treatments, or may prohibit patients from going to specialty hospitals for treatment.[24,46,47] Utilization review, preapprovals and other practice oversights may serve to overrule informed patient and physician choices. And finally, many health insurance programs fail to cover many services, especially preventive services, limiting the patient's choice and utilization of those services, even when they are efficacious and cost-effective.

A second flaw of the current system is that it lacks a systematic mechanism for assessing and informing patients about the competence of their health care delivery system and personal physician. There are few reliable and validated measures of physician and health care quality.[48,49] Medical licensure is only an indicator of minimum standards of proficiency. Specialty board examinations indicate attainment of specialized knowledge and skills beyond those required for safe practice;[50] they do not, however, provide an assessment of competence over time.[51] Hospital staff privileges are subject to review by peers and regulatory bodies. Unfortunately, their decisions tend to be influenced by politics as much as competence. Further, information about a physician's performance is not easily available to patients. Appointments to a medical faculty provide an informal system for evaluating competence, but the criteria for these appointments emphasize research, publications and other factors not necessarily associated with clinical competence. Personal recommendations and reviews of physicians in the popular press are based more on word of mouth by nonprofessionals than on reliable standards of competence. While most U.S. physicians have a good fund of knowledge and sound clinical judgment, the system fails to provide an assurance of competence. Thus, even for the best-insured Americans, the current system fails to provide reliable assessments of physician competence. Patients are left to rely on subjective impressions and reputations, neither of which are adequate.

Third, the current system contains and perpetuates threats to good communication and compassionate care. The emphasis on specialization and technical expertise and the limited training in humanistic care, communication skills and ethical considerations tend to produce physicians rooted in communication skills.[52-54] Under the threat of malpractice litigation, physicians may be inclined to order more interventions than they think are warranted.[55-57] Financial incentives in the current system encourage physicians to offer high-technology procedures rather than primary and preventive care.

The Effects of Managed Care on the Physician-Patient Relationship	
Potential Improvements	**Potential Threats**
Choice	
• Expanded choice of managed care plans, particularly in areas with low managed care penetration • Expanded choice of prevenitive and pediatric services	• "Cherry picking" increasing the number of uninsured Americans • Employers restricting patients' choice of managed care plans and physicians • Price competition forcing patients to choose between continuing with their current physicians or switching to a cheaper plan • Financial failures of managed care plans forcing change in managed care plan without choice • Restrictions by managed care plans of choice of specialists and particular services
Competence	
• Development and use of measures to assess quality of physicians and managed care plans • Greater use of preventive medical care	• Underutilization of specialists and specialized facilities • Unreliable and nonrisk-adjusted quality measures providing a distorted view of competence
Compassion	
• Increased number of generalists and primary care providers • Creation of physician – nonphysician provider teams to provide a broader range of providers knowledgeable about the patient's condition	• Productivity requirements creating shorter office visits, reduced telephone access, and other access barriers to physicians • Advertising creating inflated patient expectations
Continuity	
	• Price competition forcing patient choice of continuity at a higher price vs the cheapest plan • "Deselection" of physicians disrupting existing physician-patient relations
(No) Conflict of Interest	
	• Linking physician salary incentives and bonuses to reduced use of tests and procedures for patients

There are disincentives to talking with patients. Indeed, this is the paradigm of nonreimbursable care. In addition, bureaucratic demands for preprocedure permission, postprocedure justification, multiple reimbursement forms, and other administrative requirements take up significant physician time that might otherwise be spent discussing present and future care plans with patients.[58] Physicians may be forced to see more patients and shorten each visit so they can cover the mounting administrative personnel costs created by the explosion of paperwork.

When companies require their employees to select physicians from a restricted list, workers may be forced to change their physician.[23] Similarly, annual shifts in the cheapest managed care plan offered by a company can create a dilemma for workers as to whether continuity of care with a specific physician is worth the extra price. One recent survey found that 40% of patients in health maintenance organizations (HMOs) had to change doctors when they joined the HMO.[23] Another study found that almost half of all patients in

HMOs had been with their physician for fewer than four years, and patients in HMOs had been with their physician for a shorter period of time than patients in fee-for-service settings.[24] Thus, even for the insured American, choice and continuity of care may be, or become, an elusive ideal.

Finally, there is significant potential, if not actual, conflict of interest in the current system.[38,39,59] Physicians who practice in a fee-for-service setting and who invest in radiological or other service centers often gain financially by ordering tests and performing procedures that may not always be in the patient's best interest.[32,39,60] Conversely, physicians who practice in managed care settings may gain financially by ordering fewer tests and performing fewer procedures than is appropriate.[39,40] While the current system has implemented some rules to reduce this financial conflict of interest,[37] these rules have many defects and do not ensure no conflict of interest.[38-41]

THE PHYSICIAN-PATIENT RELATIONSHIP IN THE ERA OF MANAGED CARE

Despite the lack of comprehensive health care system reform legislation, significant changes are occurring without legislative and governmental regulation, driven predominantly by the increased efforts of employers to reduce health care costs. These changes include more managed care, increased use of primary care physicians and generalists, rather than specialists, increased use of nonphysician providers, emphasis on preventive measures, greater commitment to the care of children, and intensive quality assessment.[61,62] Although it is impossible to predict the precise concrete manifestations and effects of all these changes, it is possible to provide some educated reflections on their probable implications for the physician-patient relationship (Table). Because the health care system is so complex, the changes may not always tend in a coherent direction; some aspects may enhance a particular element of the physician-patient relationship, while others undermine it. It is often difficult to know which tendency will dominate in practice, and so we try to outline the potential trends in both directions.

Admittedly, these predictions are speculative. But they are no more speculative than projections on the cost of certain changes or on the economic consequences of particular managed care programs.[63] And just as economic projections, with uncertainty, are essential in evaluating health care proposals, so too we hope these predictions will provide a basis for planning and promoting those parts of the trend toward managed care that enhance the ideal physician-patient relationship, anticipating threats to the ideal posed by managed care, and acting to mitigate the ill-effects.

Potential Improvements

With some expansion of managed care, the range of choice for many insured Americans could also increase. Americans who live in regions without significant managed care penetration, such as the South, will soon have the option of care in a managed care setting. In addition, other Americans could now have several managed care plans, as well as fee-for-service options to choose from. However, if managed care expands too much, it may threaten to eliminate fee-for-service practitioners in a region altogether, as it appears to be doing in northern California and Minnesota. Under such circumstances, patients' choice of practice setting, even for well-insured Americans, could be effectively reduced.

Managed care may also provide the insured with a wider range of treatment alternatives. For example, by removing financial barriers, managed care plans should give enrollees more effective choice over utilizing preventive interventions, such as screening tests. Indeed, studies consistently demonstrate greater use of preventive tests and procedures among managed care enrollees.[64-66] In addition, many managed care plans contain benefits packages that include services not currently covered by many insurance programs. Indeed, pediatric patients may significantly benefit from the coverage of vaccinations, small copayments for well-child visits, and coverage of dental and visual services for children.

Managed care plans are increasingly attempting to develop quality measures; they are trying to use these quality measures for routine assessments of performance and to provide the public with the performance results based on these quality indicators. While such extensive efforts at quality assessment in medicine have never before been undertaken, and there is skepticism that these measures will be reliable and valid, if this effort is successful, many Americans will have a rigorous and systematic mechanism to evaluate the competence of their health plans and physicians.[48,49]

Besides closer monitoring of quality, other changes could improve physicians' competence and their communication with patients. The pressure created by cost controls, the resource-based relative value scale, and managed care has resulted in trends to improve reimbursement for primary care and to train more generalists. Although these initiatives are untested, they could increase the number of generalists, prompt the retraining of specialists in general medicine, and decrease the excessive reliance on specialists, with their tendency toward higher use of diagnostic tests and technical interventions without notable effect on traditional health status measures.[67-68] In addition, managed care's increased emphasis on primary care will accelerate the trend toward greater use of nurse practitioners, physician assistants, midwives and teams composed of physicians and nonphysician providers. While the transition to such a team approach could not be accomplished instantaneously, and while it would require changing habits and increased communications among health care providers, research demonstrates that, when it is well-implemented, it can improve patient care, communication and satisfactions.[69-71] With such multidisciplinary teams, several providers are knowledgeable about the patient's condition and are available to the patient, enhancing communication and continuity of care.[69,70] By increasing the number of providers for a patient, this team approach may increase the chances that patients with different cultural backgrounds might establish rapport and understanding with a provider.[69,70]

Potential Threats

There are aspects of managed care, especially under significant cost controls and price competition, with the potential to undermine, or preclude the realization of, the ideal physician-patient relationship. The spread of managed care is being promoted by big employers and corporations; it is closely linked to price competition – if not outright managed competition – which has ramifications for almost every facet of the ideal physician patient-interaction.

First, to hold down costs, many insurance companies and managed care organizations may try to select enrollees who are likely to use fewer and cheaper services ("cherry pick") through selective marketing, increased use of exclusions, modifications of benefits offered, and other techniques. In the absence of significant health insurance regulatory reform legislation or universal coverage, such techniques could mean that more Americans will be unable to afford health insurance or effectively barred from coverage. Indeed, recent statistics suggest that the ranks of the uninsured are growing.[72] In turn, this deprives more Americans of the ideal physician-patient relationship. In addition, without insurance reform legislation to ensure transportability of health coverage when people change jobs, a significant number of Americans could be forced either to forgo coverage for periods of time or to change managed care plans with each job change. Given that 7 million Americans change jobs or become employed each month, there could be significant disruption of choice, communication and continuity.

Second, to restrain costs, a growing number of employers are restricting patient choice in all its facets.[23,73-76] An increasing number of employers are offering only one health care plan; other employers are requiring their workers to enroll in a particular managed care plan or select a physician from a precertified list; still others are requiring their workers to pay substantially more for the opportunity to see a physician of their choosing outside their managed care panel; and still others are discouraging workers from selecting higher priced health plans. Some employers are even reverting to an old practice of hiring their own "company" physicians.[76] Through these and other techniques, a growing, albeit unknown, number of insured Americans are having their choice limited mainly by employers.[23] These practices may seriously disrupt, or require patients to abandon, long-standing relationships with physicians. In addition, in some instances, especially in managed care settings, patient choice of specialists, specialty facilities and particular treatments is being eroded.[24]

Increasingly, managed care plans will compete for employers' contracts and subscribers on the basis of price. Yet there is no guarantee that the cheapest plan this year will be the cheapest plan during the next enrollment period. Indeed, if price competition is effective, the cheapest plan should change from year to year.[77]

In such a price-competitive marketplace, employers may switch health care plans from year to year, and patients may be forced to choose between continuing with their current physician and managed care plan at a higher price or switching to the cheaper plan. While patients may appear to opt for discontinuous care rather than pay more, the cost pressures – which fall disproportionately on those with lower incomes – hardly make such choices voluntary.[78-80] A recent study demonstrates a direct linear relationship between a lower family income and willingness to switch to cheaper health care plans.[23] The importance of such decisions lies in the reason for change of physician.[77] Change is harmful if it is imposed on patients explicitly or implicitly by financial incentives and interrupts continuity. When the patient, however, decides to switch physicians, continuity of care has been outweighed in the patient's mind by other factors, such as competence or communication. Consequently, significant price competition, while not engendered by managed care, is certainly exacerbated by it and could have an adverse effect on both patient choice of practice type and physician and continuity of care.[23,77]

A third threat to choice in the physician-patient relationship comes from the potential financial failure of managed care plans. If price competition is effective, inefficient plans will lose in the marketplace and close. Plan failure could pose a serious threat to patient choice and continuity of care, especially if the collapse happens between enrollment periods. Under such conditions, patients may be randomly assigned to other managed care plans. Or their former physician may become affiliated with a plan that they are unable to join. Another threat to the physician-patient relationship may occur when managed care plans "deselect" a physician. In such circumstances, patients cannot choose that physician unless they are willing to go out of the plan. More important, patients who have been receiving care from that physician may be forced to switch to another physician in the managed care panel, again undermining patient choice and continuity of care.

Managed care also poses potential threats to competence. Its greater emphasis on the provision of primary care could adversely affect competence. Since specialists are more expensive than generalists, cost considerations foster a tendency to have generalists or even nonphysicians manage conditions that are best handled by specialists. For example, follow-up of cancer patients may be shifted from oncologists to primary care physicians. And there is some suggestion that these changes lead to fewer follow-up visits and less monitoring of the progress of disease in the managed setting.[81] In addition, since time spent with specialists is expensive, there may be a tendency to use medications or other less expensive interventions in place of consultations with specialists.[82] Similarly, given the current shortage of generalists, there is already a movement to retrain specialist physicians as generalists. Since there are no standards for the amount and type of education needed for retraining, these retrained specialists may lack the breadth of knowledge, skills and experience necessary to be competent primary care providers. Assessments of quality outcomes may be insensitive to these threats to competence.[83]

There are worries about the development of quality indicators. We lack quality indicators for most aspects of medical care. In addition, many quality indicators require risk adjustments for severity of illness that cannot be, or currently are not being, performed.[83,84] It will take significant time and resources to develop reliable and validated quality indicators and risk adjustors for medical procedures. Yet the demand for these indicators could result in a rush for implementation without proper pretesting and validation. Mistakes related to the imperative to release of Medicare hospital mortality data as a quality measure before they were properly adjusted may be repeated on an even larger scale.[85-88] Use of faulty quality information could damage attempts to improve the competence of physicians, undermine patient trust, and cause patients to switch physicians unnecessarily.

Communication in the physician-patient relationship could be undetermined by practice efficiencies necessitated by intensified price competition and financial pressures on managed care plans. Productivity requirements may translate into pressure on physicians to see more patients in shorter time periods, reducing the time to discuss patient values, alternative treatments, or the impact of a therapy on the patient's overall life.[89,90] Such changes have been tried by managed care plans in the competitive Boston, Mass. health care market.[91] Compressing physician-patient interactions into short time periods in the name of productivity could curtail, if not eliminate, productive communication and compassion. A recent survey of patients in managed care plans showed that the physician spent less time with the patient and offered less explanation of care compared with those in traditional fee-for-service settings.[24] Similarly, to reduce costs, managed care plans might restrict telephone calls to the patient's primary care physician. Currently, some plans limit patients' calls to their physicians to one-hour time periods in the day. In addition, incentives might be put into place to encourage patients to talk with or see physicians or nonphysician providers with whom they are unfamiliar or who are not of their choosing.[82,90] All of these cost-saving mechanisms could easily inhibit physician-patient communication and continuity of care.

A further problem may arise in the competition among managed care plans to lure subscribers. They are likely to use advertising with implicit, if not explicit, promises of higher quality or more wide-ranging services. Such advertisements could easily create high expectations on the part of patients.[92-94] Simultaneously, however, to control costs plans will require physicians to be efficient in their personal time allocation as well as in their ordering of tests and use of other services. This could easily create a conflict between patient expectations and physician restrictions, under good communication, compassion and trust.

Finally, while there has been significant attention on conflict of interest in fee-for-service practice,[39] there has been much less effort to investigate and address conflict of interest in managed care. Physician decision-making may account for as much as 75% of health care costs. In the setting of significant price competition, managed care plans trying to reduce costs will therefore try to influence physician decision-making, especially to reduce the use of medical services.[89] Managed care plans have already tried various mechanisms to try to reduce physician use of health care resources for their patients, including providing bonuses to physicians who order few tests and basing a percentage of physicians' salaries on volume and test ordering standards.[39,40,89] Such conflicts of interest may proliferate with increased price competition, the need for managed care plans to reduce costs, and the absence of governmental regulation.

CONCLUSIONS

The physician-patient relationship is the cornerstone for achieving, maintaining and improving health. The structure of financing and regulation should be designed to foster and support an ideal relationship between the physician and the patient. Clearly, the current system incompletely realizes this ideal even for many well-insured Americans, and trends within the current system threaten to make its ideal even more elusive.

Managed care offers some advantages in realizing the ideal physician-patient relationship. For many Americans, increased use of managed care may secure choice, especially for preventive services, possibly expand continuity in their relationship with physicians, and implement a systematic assessment of quality and competence. But the expansion of managed care, in an environment that encourages competition and makes financial pressures intense and omnipresent, could promote serious impediments to realizing the ideal physician-patient relationship. Some practical steps that might diminish these impediments include (1) using global budgets instead of price competition among managed care plans for cost control; (2) prohibiting all schemes that use salary incentives or bonuses tied to physician test-ordering patterns; (3) restricting expensive advertising by managed care plans by capping their promotion budgets; (4) requiring managed care plans to have a board of patients and physicians to approve policies regarding length of office visits and telephone calls; (5) creating an independent review board to assess the reliability and validity of all quality indicators before they are approved or required for use by managed care plans; (6) implementing insurance reform legislation to ensure mobility of insurance with job changes and purchasing of coverage by individuals; and (7) providing universal coverage to enable otherwise uninsured patients to have an opportunity for an ideal physician-patient relationship. As changes in our health care system develop, we must find ways, such as these, to encourage fiscal prudence without undermining the fundamental elements of the ideal physician-patient relationship.

KEY IDEAS IN THIS ARTICLE:

- "The physician-patient relationship is the cornerstone for achieving, maintaining and improving health. The structure of financing and regulation should be designed to foster and support an ideal relationship between the physician and the patient."

- "To evaluate the effects of managed care, we need to delineate an ideal conception of the physician-patient relationship."

- "We suggest that the fundamental elements of the ideal physician-patient relationship that are embodied in our intuitions and common to ethical analyses and legal standards can be expressed as six C's: choice, competence, communication, compassion, continuity, and (no) conflict of interest."

- "Four critical elements of *choice* are: 1) choice of practice type and setting; 2) choice of primary care physician; 3) choice of a specialist or special facility in an emergency or for a special condition; 4) choice among treatment alternatives."

- *Competence* includes: 1) a good fund of knowledge kept current; 2) good diagnostic and treatment skills; 3) good clinical judgment for fine-grained differentiation; 4) knowledge and acceptance of their own limitations.

- *Communication* includes: 1) ability to listen and grasp patient concerns and values; 2) enhancing patients' ability to articulate and helping patients identify the limits, if any, of their desire for knowledge; 3) communicating in language accessible to patients and relating technical data to patient values.

- *Compassion* means that patients experience their world of concerns and values as: 1) important; 2) understood; 3) central in determining the care they receive.

- *Continuity* provides the extended time and evolution of relationship that is necessary for the other essential elements to have their full impact on the health of the patient.

- *(No) Conflict of interest* means that "we expect that a physician's primary concern will be his or her patient's well-being, even though physicians may have obligations that conflict."

- Some practical steps that might diminish the impediments include:

  1) using global budgets instead of price competition among managed care plans for cost control;

  2) prohibiting all schemes that use salary incentives or bonuses tied to physician test-ordering patterns;

  3) restricting expensive advertising by managed care plans by capping their promotion budgets;

  4) requiring managed care plans to have a board of patients and physicians to approve policies regarding length of office visits and telephone calls;

  5) creating an independent review board to assess the reliability and validity of all quality indicators before they are approved or required for use by managed care plans;

  6) implementing insurance reform legislation to ensure mobility of insurance with job changes and purchasing of coverage by individuals;

  7) providing universal coverage to enable otherwise uninsured patients to have an opportunity for an ideal physician-patient relationship.

A SUGGESTED PROCESS FOR REFLECTING ON THIS ARTICLE:

(see pages 234-254 for other processes that might better fit your specific goals and objectives).

The authors suggest six key elements of the ideal physician-patient relationship that should be considered. In the grid below, construct your own list of essential elements of the ideal physician-patient relationship, adapting their elements as you see fit and ranking their relative importance.

✓ if one of your key elements		Importance 1-5 5=high
	Choice	
	Competence	
	Communication	
	Compassion	
	Continuity	
	(No) Conflict of Interest	
	other _____	
	other _____	
	other _____	

In column A, list your essential elements of the ideal physician-patient relationship.

In column B, indicate how fee-for-service can enhance this element.

In column C, indicate how fee-for-service can diminish this element.

In column D, indicate how managed care can enhance this element.

In column E, indicate how managed care can diminish this element.

A Essentials of ideal physician-patientrelationship	B FFS +	C FFS-	D Mgd Care +	E Mgd Care
1				
2				
3				
4				
5				
6				
7				
8				
9				

IN LIGHT OF OUR DISCUSSION:

- as (executive committee, ethics committee, etc.) what are some next steps that we should take?

- as (hospital, home health agency, etc.), what are some next steps that we should take?

- what systems and structures call for special attention in order to improve the situation?

ENDNOTES

1. Miller RH, Luft HS. Managed care plan performance since 1980. *JAMA* 1994:271:1512-1519.

2. Schwartz WB, Mendelson DN. Why managed care cannot contain hospital costs – without rationing. *Health Aff* (Millwood). 1992;11:100-107.

3. Moran DW, Wolfe PR. Can managed care control costs? *Health Aff* (Millwood). 1991;10:120-128.

4. Fox PD, Wasserman J. Academic medical centers and managed care. *Health Aff* (Millwood), 1993; 12:85-93.

5. Eckholm E. A town loses its hospital in the name of cost control. *New York Times.* September 26, 1994:Al.

6. Weber M. The fundamental concepts of sociology. In: Parsons T, ed. *The Theory of Social and Economic Organization.* New York, NY: The Free Press; 1947:87-157.

7. Macklin R. *Enemies of Patients.* New York, NY: Oxford University Press Inc; 1993:chaps 1, 5, 7, 11.

8. Brody H. *The Healer's Power.* New Haven, Conn: Yale University Press; 1992:chaps 4-8.

9. Emanuel EJ, Emanuel LL. Four models of the physician-patient relationship. *JAMA.* 1992;267:2221-2226.

10. Brock D. The ideal of shared decision-making between physicians and patients. *Kennedy Inst J Ethics.* 1991;1:28-47.

11. Campbell JD, Mauksch HO, Meikirk HJ, Hosokawa MC. Collaborative practice and provider styles of delivering health care. *Soc Sci Med. 1990;* 30:1359-1385.

12. Beauchamp T, Childress J. *Principles of Biomedical Ethics.* 3rd ed. New York, NY: Oxford University Press; 1989:chaps 3-5, 7.

13. Kass LR. *Toward a More Natural Science.* New York. NY: The Free Press; 1988:chaps 6-9.

14. Appelbaum PS, Lidz C, Meisel A. *Informed Consent: Legal Theory and Clinical Practice.* New York, NY: Oxford University Press Inc; 1987.

15. Siegler M. The profession of medicine: from physician paternalism to patient autonomy to bureaucratic parsimony. *Arch Intern Med.* 1985;145: 713-715.

16. Katz J. *The Silent World of Doctor and Patient.* New York, NY: The Free Press; 1984.

17. *Making Health Care Decisions.* Washington, DC: President's Commission for the Study of Ethical Problems in Medicine and Biomedical and Behavioral Research; 1982.

18. Veatch RM. *A Theory of Medical Ethics.* New York, NY: Basic Books Inc Publishers; 1980:pts 2 and 3.

19. Szasz TS, Hollender MH. The basic models of the doctor-patient relationship. *Arch Intern Med.* 1956;97:585-592.

20. Rawls J. *Political Liberalism.* New York, NY: Columbia University Press; 1993;pt 1.

21. Dworkin R. *Taking Rights Seriously.* Cambridge, Mass: Harvard University Press; 1977:Chaps 2-4.

22. Emanuel EJ. *The Ends of Human Life: Medical Ethics in a Liberal Polity.* Cambridge, Harvard University Press; 1991:Chap 1.

23. *The Kaiser/Commonwealth Fund Second National Health Insurance Survey.* November 10, 1993.

24. Blendon RJ, Knox RA, Brodie M, Benson JM, Chervinsky G. Americans compare managed care, Medicare, and fee for service. *J Am Health Policy.* 1994;4:42-47.

25. Sofaer S. Informing and protecting consumers under managed competition. *Health Aff* (Millwood). 1993;12 (suppl):76-86.

26. Ingelfinger FJ. "Arrogance." *N. Eng. J. Med.* 1980; 304:1507.

27. Marzuk PM. The right kind of paternalism. *N. Engl. J. Med.* 1985;313:1474-1476.

28. Applegate WB. Physician management of patients with adverse outcomes. *Arch Intern Med.* 1986;146:2249-2252.

29. Ware J, Snyder M. Dimensions of patient attitudes regarding doctors and medical services. *Med Care.* 1975;13:669-682.

30. Woofley FR, Kane RL, Hughes CC, Wright DD. The effects of doctor-patient communication on satisfaction and outcome of care. *Soc Sci Med.* 1978;12:123-128.

31. Hickson GB, Clayton EW, Githens PB, Sloan FA. Factors that prompted families to file medical malpractice claims following perinatal injuries. *JAMA,* 1992;267:1359-1363.

32. Feilich B. The death of a baby: neither forgiven nor forgotten. *JAMA* 1992;268:1413-1414.

33. Spiro H, McCrea-Curnen MG, Peschel I, St. James D, eds. *Empathy and the Practice of Medicine.* New Haven, Conn: Yale University Press; 1993: chaps 1-3, 8, 9, 13-16.

34. Jonsen A. *The New Medicine and the Old Ethics.* Cambridge, Mass: Harvard University Press; 1990.

35. *Tarasoff v Regents of the University of California et al,* 131 Cal Rptr 14 (1976).

36. *McIntosh v Milano,* 168 NJ 466 (1979).

37. Council on Ethical and Judicial Affairs, American Medical Association. Conflict of interest: physician ownership of medical facilities. *JAMA* 1992; 267:2366-2369.

38. Thompson D. Understanding financial conflicts of interest. *N. Engl. J. Med.* 1993;329:573-576.

39. Rodwin M. *Medicine, Money, and Morals.* New York, NY: Oxford University Press Inc; 1993.

40. Hillman AL, Pauly MV, Kerstein JJ. How do financial incentives affect physicians' clinical decisions and the financial performance of health maintenance organizations? *N. Engl. J. Med.* 1989;321:86-92.

41. Relman AS. Dealing with conflicts of interest. *N. Engl. J. Med.,* 1985;313:749-751.

42. Nelson C, Short K. *Health Insurance Coverage, 1986-88.* Washington, DC: US Bureau of the Census; 1990.

43. Lewin-Epstein N. Determinants of regular source of health care in black, Mexican, Puerto Rican, and non-Hispanic white populations. *Med. Care.* 1991;29:543-557.

44. Hadley J, Steinberg EP, Feder J. Comparison of uninsured and privately insured hospital patients: condition on admission, resource use, and outcome. *JAMA* 1991:265:374-379.

45. Burstin HR, Lipsitz SR, Brennan TA. Socioeconomic status and risk for substandard medical care. *JAMA* 1992;268:2383-2387.

46. Iglehart JK. The American health care system: teaching hospitals. *N. Eng. J. Med.* 1993:329:1052-1056.

47. Hoch S. Tsongas's case. *New York Times.* February 20, 1992:A23.

48. Laffel G, Berwick DM. Quality in health care. *JAMA.* 1992:407-409.

49. Kritchevsky SB, Simmons BP. Continuous quality improvement: concepts and applications for physician care. *JAMA* 1991;266:1817-1823.

50. Ramsey PG, Carline JD, Inui TS, Larson EB, LoGerfo JP, Wenrich MD. Predictive validity of certification by the American Board of Internal Medicine. *Ann Intern Med.* 1989;110:719-726.

51. Benson JA.Certification and recertification:one approach to professional accountability. *Ann Intern Med.* 1991;114:238-242.

52. Merkel WT, Margolis RB, 5th RC. Teaching humanistic and psychosocial aspects of care. *J Gen Intern Med.* 1990;5:34-41.

53. Beckman H, Frankel R, Kihm J, Kulesza G, Geheb M. Measurement and improvement of humanistic skills in first year trainees. *J Gen Intern Med.* 1990;5:42-45.

54. Levinson W, Roter D. The effects of two continuing medical education programs on communication skills of practicing primary care physicians. *J Gen Intern Med.* 1993;8:318-324.

55. Perkins HS, Bauer RL, Hazuda HP, Schoolfield JD. Impact of legal liability, family wishes, and other "external factors" on physicians' life support decisions. *Am J Med.* 1990;89:185-194.

56. Localio AR, Lawthers AG, Bengtson JM, et al. Relationship between malpractice claims and cesarean delivery. *JAMA* 1993;269:366-373.

57. Rosenbach ML, Stone AG. Malpractice insurance costs and physician practice 1983-1986. *Health Aff* (Millwood). 1990;9:176-185.

58. Woolhandler S, Himmelstein D. The deteriorating administrative efficiency of the U.S. health care system. *N Engl J Med.* 1991;324:1253-1258.

59. Gray B. *The Profit Motive and Patient Care.* Cambridge, Mass: Harvard University Press; 1991: chaps 5-8, 10, 11.

60. Mitchell JM, Scott E. Physician ownership of physical therapy services: effects on charges, utilization, profits, and service characteristics. *JAMA.* 1992;268:2055.

61. Igelhart JK. The struggle between managed care and fee for service practice. *N. Engl. J. Med.* 1994;331:63-67.

62. *Effects of Managed Care: An Update.* Washington, DC: Congressional Budget Office; 1994.

63. *Managed Health Care: Effects on Employers' Costs Difficult to Measure.* Washington, DC: US General Accounting Office; 1993.

64. Bernstein AB, Thompson GB, Harlan LC. Differences in rates of cancer screening by usual source of medical care: data from the 1987 National Health Interview Survey. *Med Care.* 1991;29:196-209.

65. Retchin SM, Brown B. The quality of ambulatory care in Medicare health maintenance organizations. *Am J Public Health.* 1990;80:411-415.

66. Udvarhelyi IS, Jennison K, Phillips RS, Epstein AM. Comparison of the quality of ambulatory care for fee-for-service and prepaid patients. *Ann Intern Med.* 1991;327:424.

67. Greenfield S., Nelson EC, Zubkoff M, et al. Variations in resource utilization among medical specialties and systems of care. *JAMA.* 1992;267:1624-1630.

68. Schroder SA, Sandy LG. Specialty distribution of U.S. physicians – the invisible driver of health care costs. *N. Engl. J. Med.* 1993;328:961-963.

69. *Nurse Practitioners, Physicians' Assistants, and Certified Nurse Midwives: Policy Analysis.* Washington, DC: Office of Technology Assessment; 1986.

70. Freund C. Research in support of nurse practitioners. In: Mezey M, McGivern D, eds. *Nurses and Nurse Practitioners: The Evolution to Advanced Practice.* New York, NY: Springer Publishing Co Inc: 1993.

71. Kavesh W. Physician and nurse-practitioner relationships. In: Mezey M, McGivern D, eds. *Nurses and Nurse Practitioners: The Evolution to Advanced Practice.* New York, NY: Springer Publishing Co., Inc; 1993.

72. Pear R. Health insurance percentage is lowest in four Sun Belt states. *New York Times.* October 6, 1994:A16.

73. Lewis DE. Coping without coverage. *Boston Globe*. May 5, 1993:45.

74. Lewis DE. Union oks Boston gas accord. *Boston Globe*. May 21, 1993:53.

75. Seitz R. The political tea leaves point to medical networks. *New York Times*. December 20,1992:D10.

76. Pasternak J. In-house doctors give some firms a health care remedy. *Los Angeles Times*. July 11, 1993:Al.

77. Emanuel EJ, Brett AS. Managed competition and the patient-physician relationship. *N Engl J Med*. 1993;329:879-882.

78. Travis MR, Russell G, Cronin S. "Determinants of voluntary disenrollment." *J Health Care Marketing*. 1989;9:75-76.

79. Hennely VD, Boxerman SB. Out-of-plan use and disenrollment: outgrowths of dissatisfaction with a prepaid group plan. *Med Care*. 1983;21:348-359.

80. Sorenson AA, Wersinger RP. Factors influencing disenrollment from an HMO. *Med Care*. 1981;19:766-773.

81. Clement DG, Retchin SM, Brown RS, Stegall MH. Access and outcomes of elderly patients enrolled in managed care. *JAMA*. 1994;271:1487-1492.

82. Henneberger M. Managed changing practice of psychotherapy. *New York Times*. October 9, 1994:Al, A50.

83. Salem-Schatz S, Moore G, Rucker M, Pearson SD. The case for case-mix adjustment in practice profiling when good apples look bad. *JAMA* 1994;272:871-874.

84. McNeil BJ, Pederson SH, Gatsonis C. Current issues in profiling quality of care. *Inquiry*. 1992;299:298-307.

85. Green J, Passman LJ, Wintfield N. Analyzing hospital mortality: the consequences of diversity in patient mix. *JAMA* 1991;265:1849-1853.

86. Burke M. HCFA's Medicare mortality data: the controversy continues. *Hospitals*. 1992:118, 120, 122.

87. Greenfield S. Aronow HU, Elashoff RM, Wantanabe D. Flaws in mortality data: the hazards of ignoring comorbid disease. *JAMA* 1988;260:2253-2255.

88. Robinson ML. Limitations of mortality data confirmed: studies. *Hospitals*. 1988;62:23-24.

89. Baker LC, Cantor JC. Physician satisfaction under managed care. *Health Aff* (Millwood). 1993; 122 (suppl):258-270.

90. Jellinek MS, Nurcombe B. Two wrongs don't make a right: managed care, mental health, and the marketplace. *JAMA*. 1993;270:1737-1739.

91. Knox RA, Stein C. HMO doctors want boss out in dispute on patient load. *Boston Globe*. November 21, 1991:1, 27.

92. Freidson E. Prepaid group practice and the new 'demanding patients.' *Milbank Mem Fund Q*. 1973;51:473-488.

93. Schroeder JL, Clarke JT, Webster JR. Prepaid entitlements:a new challenge for physician-patient relationships. *JAMA*. 1985;254:3080-3082.

94. Brett AS. The case against persuasive advertising by health maintenance organizations. *N. Engl. J. Med*. 1992;326:1253-1257.

PART 4

PROCESSING KEY IDEAS AND
PROCESSES FOR REFLECTION AND ACTION

CHAPTER 18

10 METHODS FOR PROCESSING KEY IDEAS

INTRODUCTION

What is your goal for this discussion?

If you don't care where you are going, any road will get you there. This is true for processing in a group. Simply opening up a discussion of a complex issue with "what do you think about . . .?" ususally results in a disjointed and frustrating conversation. But even thorny issues can be handled in a rewarding and productive way if we are clear and realistic about out objectives for a discussion and put a process in place to meet such objections. We can engage a group in reflection for a wide range of reasons. A partial list of such reasons includes:

- to engage in shared learning
- to share information
- to debate
- to develop policy
- to make a decision
- to set goals
- to develop strategies
- to manage conflict
- to identify problems
- to solve problems
- to clarify values
- to build community/team
- to develop consensus
- to explore diverse opinions
- to examine our organization's systems and structures
- to generate creativity
- to assess and evaluate

Effective discussion does not happen by accident. The longer range our goals and more expansive our hopes, the more important it is to think of this the way we think of building a big and expensive new facility.

Here's a checklist of some issues that can help plan discussion:

GOALS: • long range • short range • primary • secondary	
Timeframe: • long range • short range	
Key elements of larger process:	
Key elements of this specific process:	
Key elements: • send out article/survey? • collate results? • send out results?	
Handouts needed:	
Space needed:	
Equipment:	

10 PROCESSES FOR DISCUSSING ONE ARTICLE

The following 10 processes show how the same article could be used in different ways, depending on the purpose one has for engaging the group in discussion of the material.

MAKING THE CASE FOR NOT-FOR-PROFIT HEALTHCARE:
Cardinal Joseph Bernardin

Key ideas in this article include:

1. A good society needs both economic goods (cars, toasters, computers, etc.) and noneconomic goods (families, education, healthcare, etc.). It should treat these different goods in essentially different ways.

2. There are two different kinds of social institutions: 1) those whose primary purpose is to earn a profit and reasonable rate of return on investment; 2) those whose primary purpose is to advance human dignity (family, schools, courts, cities, etc.).

3. "The idea that the entirety of social life is to be determined by market exchanges is to run 'the risk of an idolatry of the market, an idolatry which ignores the existence of goods which by their nature are not and cannot be mere commodities.' "

4. "The purpose of a not-for-profit organization is to improve the human condition, that is, to advance important noneconomic, nonregulatory functions that cannot be as well-served by either business corporations or government."

5. "The primary question in an investor-owned organization is: How do we ensure a reasonable return to our shareholders? Other questions may be asked . . . but always in the context of their effect on profit."

6. Four essential characteristics of healthcare delivery are especially compatible with not-for-profit structure:

   a) Access: "With primary accountability to shareholders, investor-owned organizations have a powerful incentive to avoid uninsured . . . hard-to-serve, high-cost populations . . . undesirable geographic . . . low-density rural areas."

   b) Patient-first ethic: "Not-for-profit healthcare organizations are better suited than their investor-owned counterparts to support the patient-first ethic in medicine."

   c) Community-wide needs: "In healthcare there are a host of community-wide needs that are generally unprofitable, and therefore unlikely to be addressed by investor-owned organizations."

   d) Volunteerism: "Volunteerism and philanthropy are important components of healthcare that thrive best in a not-for-profit setting."

7. Besides business and government, we need mediating institutions (e.g., family, church, schools, healthcare facilities). Such institutions stand between large, bureaucratic government and the individual; they also mediate against the rougher edges of capitalism's inclination toward excessive individualism. The character of not-for-profit healthcare is more compatible with effective mediating institutions.

8. "Private and public sector leaders have an urgent civic responsibility to preserve and strengthen our nation's predominantly not-for-profit healthcare delivery system."

10 PROCESSES FOR DISCUSSING ONE ARTICLE: PROCESS 1

Purpose: To get the group to take a position on each of the key ideas of the article and share this information with the whole group.

The following questionnaire could be used in several ways:

1) It could be sent out ahead of time with the article, filled out, sent back and collated with the graphed responses, serving as the basis for a discussion.

2) It could be sent out ahead of time with the article and each participant could come with their completed questionnaire, prepared to discuss their responses.

1. A good society needs both economic goods (cars, toasters, computers, etc.) and noneconomic goods (families, education, healthcare, etc.). It should treat these different goods in essentially different ways.

❑ strongly agree ❑ agree ❑ not sure ❑ disagree ❑ strongly disagree
Comment:

2. There are two different kinds of social institutions: 1) those whose primary purpose is to earn a profit and reasonable rate of return on investment; 2) those whose primary purpose is to advance human dignity (family, schools, courts, cities, etc.).

❑ strongly agree ❑ agree ❑ not sure ❑ disagree ❑ strongly disagree
Comment:

3. "The idea that the entirety of social life is to be determined by market exchanges is to run 'the risk of an idolatry of the market, an idolatry which ignores the existence of goods which by their nature are not and cannot be mere commodities.'"

❑ strongly agree ❑ agree ❑ not sure ❑ disagree ❑ strongly disagree
Comment:

4. "The purpose of a not-for-profit organization is to improve the human condition, that is to advance important noneconomic, nonregulatory functions that cannot be as well served by either business corporations or government."

❑ strongly agree ❑ agree ❑ not sure ❑ disagree ❑ strongly disagree
Comment:

5. "The primary question in an investor-owned organization is: How do we ensure a reasonable return to our shareholders? Other questions may be asked . . . but always in the context of their effect on profit."

❑ strongly agree ❑ agree ❑ not sure ❑ disagree ❑ strongly disagree
Comment:

6. Four essential characteristics of healthcare delivery are especially compatible with not-for-profit structure.

a) Access: "With primary accountability to shareholders, investor-owned organizations have a powerful incentive to avoid uninsured . . . hard-to-serve, high-cost populations. . . undesirable geographic. . . low-density rural areas."
   ❑ strongly agree ❑ agree ❑ not sure ❑ disagree ❑ strongly disagree
   Comment:

b) Patient-first ethic: "Not-for-profit healthcare organizations are better suited than their investor-owned counterparts to support the patient-first ethic in medicine."
   ❑ strongly agree ❑ agree ❑ not sure ❑ disagree ❑ strongly disagree
   Comment:

c) Community-wide needs: "In healthcare there are a host of community-wide needs that are generally unprofitable, and therefore unlikely to be addressed by investor-owned organizations."
   ❑ strongly agree ❑ agree ❑ not sure ❑ disagree ❑ strongly disagree
   Comment:

d) Volunteerism: "Volunteerism and philanthropy are important components of healthcare that thrive best in a not-for-profit setting."
   ❑ strongly agree ❑ agree ❑ not sure ❑ disagree ❑ strongly disagree
   Comment:

7. Besides business and government, we need mediating institutions (e.g., family, church, schools, healthcare facilities). Such institutions stand between large, bureaucratic government and the individual; they also mediate against the rougher edges of capitalism's inclination toward excessive individualism. The character of not-for-profit healthcare is more compatible with effective mediating institutions.
   ❑ strongly agree ❑ agree ❑ not sure ❑ disagree ❑ strongly disagree
   Comment:

8. "Private and public sector leaders have an urgent civic responsibility to preserve and strengthen our nation's predominantly not-for-profit healthcare delivery system."

❑ strongly agree ❑ agree ❑ not sure ❑ disagree ❑ strongly disagree

Comment:

In Light of Our Discussion:

- as (executive committee, as ethics committee, etc.), what are some next steps that we should take?

- as (hospital, home health agency, etc.), what are some next steps that we should take?

- what systems and structures call for special attention in order to improve the situation?

10 PROCESSES FOR DISCUSSING ONE ARTICLE: PROCESS 2

Purpose: To provide a narrower focus on a few key ideas, with a more in-depth discussion of these select issues.

Only a select number of key ideas could be selected to provide a sharper focus and more in-depth discussion of the issues. For example, ideas 1-5 might be selected. And the focus could be in the area of intellectual understanding and agreement.

1. A good society needs both economic goods (cars, toasters, computers, etc.) and non-economic goods (families, education, healthcare, etc.). It should treat these different goods in essentially different ways.

   What makes sense to me about this is:

   What does not make sense to me about this is:

2. There are two different kinds of social institutions: 1) those whose primary purpose is to earn a profit and reasonable rate of return on investment; 2) those whose primary purpose is to advance human dignity (family, schools, courts, cities, etc.).

   What makes sense to me about this is:

   What does not make sense to me about this is:

3. "The idea that the entirety of social life is to be determined by market exchanges is to run 'the risk of an idolatry of the market, an idolatry which ignores the existence of goods which by their nature are not and cannot be mere commodities.' "

What makes sense to me about this is:

What does not make sense to me about this is:

4. "The purpose of a not-for-profit organization is to improve the human condition, that is, to advance important noneconomic, nonregulatory functions that cannot be as well-served by either business corporations or government."

What makes sense to me about this is:

What does not make sense to me about this is:

5. "The primary question in an investor-owned organization is: How do we ensure a reasonable return to our shareholders? Other questions may be asked . . . but always in the context of their effect on profit."

What makes sense to me about this is:

What does not make sense to me about this is:

In Light of Our Discussion:

- as (executive committee, ethics committee, etc.), what are some next steps that we should take?

- as (hospital, home health agency, etc.), what are some next steps that we should take?

- what systems and structures call for special attention in order to improve the situation?

10 PROCESSES FOR DISCUSSING ONE ARTICLE: PROCESS 3

Purpose: On a select number of issues, invite a more personal self-examination and sharing of personal values.

1. A good society needs both economic goods (cars, toasters, computers, etc.) and noneconomic goods (families, education, healthcare, etc.). It should

treat these different goods in essentially different ways.

This relates to some personal reasons/values/experiences that I have relative to health care.

❑ Hardly ❑ Somewhat ❑ Much

Comment:

2. There are two different kinds of social institutions: 1) those whose primary purpose is to earn a profit and reasonable rate of return on investment; 2) those whose primary purpose is to advance human dignity (family, schools, courts, cities, etc.).

This relates to some personal reasons/values/experiences that I have relative to health care.

❑ Hardly ❑ Somewhat ❑ Much

Comment:

3. "The idea that the entirety of social life is to be determined by market exchanges is to run 'the risk of an idolatry of the market, an idolatry which ignores the existence of goods which by their nature are not and cannot be mere commodities.' "

This relates to some personal reasons/values/experiences that I have relative to health care.

❑ Hardly ❑ Somewhat ❑ Much

Comment:

4. "The purpose of a not-for-profit organization is to improve the human condition, that is, to advance important noneconomic, nonregulatory functions that cannot be as well-served by either business corporations or government."

This relates to some personal reasons/values/experiences that I have relative to health care.

❑ Hardly ❑ Somewhat ❑ Much

Comment:

5. "The primary question in an investor-owned organization is: How do we ensure a reasonable return to our shareholders? Other questions may be asked . . . but always in the context of their effect on profit."

This relates to some personal reasons/values/experiences that I have relative to health care.

❑ Hardly ❑ Somewhat ❑ Much

Comment:

In light of our discussion:

- as (executive committee, ethics committee, etc.), what are some next steps that we should take?

- as (hospital, home health agency, etc.), what are some next some next steps that we should take?

- what systems and structures call for special attention in order to improve the situation?

10 PROCESSES FOR DISCUSSING ONE ARTICLE: PROCESS 4

Purpose: To examine/discuss the similarities and differences between each individual's own position and how each person judges their team's position on this issue.

I agree personally 1-5 5=high		Our mgt. team agrees 1-5 5=high
	1. A good society needs both economic goods (cars, toasters, computers, etc.) and noneconomic goods (families, education, healthcare, etc.). It should treat these different goods in essentially different ways.	
	2. There are two different kinds of social institutions: 1) those whose primary purpose is to earn a profit and reasonable rate of return on investment; 2) those whose primary purpose is to advance human dignity (family, schools, courts, cities, etc.).	
	3. "The idea that the entirety of social life is to be determined by market exchanges is to run 'the risk of an idolatry of the market, an idolatry which ignores the existence of goods which by their nature are not and cannot be mere commodities.' "	
	4. "The purpose of a not-for-profit organization is to improve the human condition, that is, to advance important noneconomic, nonregulatory functions that cannot be as well-served by either business corporations or government."	
	5. "The primary question in an investor-owned organization is: How do we ensure a reasonable return to our shareholders? Other questions may be asked . . . but always in the context of their effect on profit."	

In Light of Our Discussion:

- as (executive committee, ethics committee, etc.), what are some next steps that we should take?

- as (hospital, home health agency, etc.), what are some next steps that we should take?

- what systems and structures call for special attention in order to improve the situation?

10 PROCESSES FOR DISCUSSING ONE ARTICLE: PROCESS 5

Purpose: To examine/discuss the relationship between our organization's rhetoric and its infrastructure for accomplishing the ideals of this rhetoric.

Our org. rhetoric agrees 1-5 5=high		Our org. systems/ structures agree 1-5 5=high
	1. A good society needs both economic goods (cars, toasters, computers, etc.) and noneconomic goods (families, education, healthcare, etc.). It should treat these different goods in essentially different ways.	
	2. There are two different kinds of social institutions: 1) those whose primary purpose is to earn a profit and reasonable rate of return on investment; 2) those whose primary purpose is to advance human dignity (family, schools, courts, cities, etc.).	
	3. "The idea that the entirety of social life is to be determined by market exchanges is to run 'the risk of an idolatry of the market, an idolatry which ignores the existence of goods which by their nature are not and cannot be mere commodities.' "	
	4. "The purpose of a not-for-profit organization is to improve the human condition, that is, to advance important noneconomic, nonregulatory functions that cannot be as well served by either business corporations or government."	
	5. "The primary question in an investor-owned organization is: How do we ensure a reasonable return to our shareholders? Other questions may be asked . . . but always in the context of their effect on profit."	

In light of our discussion:

- as (executive committee, ethics committee, etc.), what are some next steps that we should take?

- as (hospital, home health agency, etc.), what are some next steps that we should take?

- what systems and structures call for special attention in order to improve the situation?

10 PROCESSES FOR DISCUSSING ONE ARTICLE: PROCESS 6

Purpose: To discuss/examine some specific areas of action that deserve attention.

	use as mgmt selection criterion 1-5 5=high	express more strongly in basic documents.	make more object of advocacy	do more in-house education	do more education of general public
1. A good society needs both economic goods (cars, toasters, computers, etc.) and noneconomic goods (families, education, healthcare, etc.). It should treat these different goods in essentially different ways.					
2. There are two different kinds of social institutions: 1) those whose primary purpose is to earn a profit and reasonable rate of return on investment; 2) those whose primary purpose is to advance human dignity (family, schools, courts, cities, etc.).					
3. "The idea that the entirety of social life is to be determined by market exchanges is to run 'the risk of an idolatry of the market, an idolatry which ignores the existence of goods which by their nature are not and cannot be mere commodities.' "					
4. "The purpose of a not-for-profit organization is to improve the human condition, that is, to advance important noneconomic, nonregulatory functions that cannot be as well-served by either business corporations or government."					
5. "The primary question in an investor-owned organization is: How do we ensure a reasonable return to our shareholders? Other questions may be asked . . . but always in the context of their effect on profit."					

In light of our discussion:

- as (executive committee, ethics committee, etc.), what are some next steps that we should take?

- as (hospital, home health agency, etc.), what are some next steps that we should take?

- what systems and structures call for special attention in order to improve the situation?

10 PROCESSES FOR DISCUSSING ONE ARTICLE: PROCESS 7

Purpose: To examine/discuss the relationship between our organization's understanding of these issues and the understanding of our larger culture.

Our org. philosophy & values agree 1-5 5=high		U.S. public agrees 1-5 5=high
	1. A good society needs both economic goods (cars, toasters, computers, etc.) and noneconomic goods (families, education, healthcare, etc.). It should treat these different goods in essentially different ways.	
	2. There are two different kinds of social institutions: 1) those whose primary purpose is to earn a profit and reasonable rate of return on investment; 2) those whose primary purpose is to advance human dignity (family, schools, courts, cities, etc.).	
	3. "The idea that the entirety of social life is to be determined by market exchanges is to run 'the risk of an idolatry of the market, an idolatry which ignores the existence of goods which by their nature are not and cannot be mere commodities.'"	
	4. "The purpose of a not-for-profit organization is to improve the human condition, that is, to advance important noneconomic, nonregulatory functions that cannot be as well-served by either business corporations or government."	
	5. "The primary question in an investor-owned organization is: How do we ensure a reasonable return to our shareholders? Other questions may be asked . . . but always in the context of their effect on profit."	

In light of our discussion:

- as (executive committee, ethics committee, etc.), what are some next steps that we should take?

- as (hospital, home health agency, etc.), what are some next steps that we should take?

- what systems and structures call for special attention in order to improve the situation?

Purpose: To take one central issue and examine it from a number of the perspectives elaborated above.

> "Private and public sector leaders have an urgent civic responsibility to preserve and strengthen our nation's predominantly not-for-profit healthcare system."

This makes sense to me personally.

❑ strongly agree ❑ agree ❑ not sure ❑ disagree ❑ strongly disagree

Our management team should have a strong consensus on this issue.
❑ strongly agree ❑ agree ❑ not sure ❑ disagree ❑ strongly disagree

Our management team does have a strong consensus on this issue.
❑ strongly agree ❑ agree ❑ not sure ❑ disagree ❑ strongly disagree

We have spelled this out clearly in our foundation documents.
❑ strongly agree ❑ agree ❑ not sure ❑ disagree ❑ strongly disagree

There is a good match between our rhetoric and our actions on this question.
❑ strongly agree ❑ agree ❑ not sure ❑ disagree ❑ strongly disagree

The governance of our entities should have a consensus on this issue.
❑ strongly agree ❑ agree ❑ not sure ❑ disagree ❑ strongly disagree

The governance of our entities does have a consensus on this issue.
❑ strongly agree ❑ agree ❑ not sure ❑ disagree ❑ strongly disagree

This should be an explicit concern in hiring or promoting persons for senior management.
❑ strongly agree ❑ agree ❑ not sure ❑ disagree ❑ strongly disagree

We should invest more resources in advocacy on this issue.
❑ strongly agree ❑ agree ❑ not sure ❑ disagree ❑ strongly disagree

We should do more internal education on this issue.
❑ strongly agree ❑ agree ❑ not sure ❑ disagree ❑ strongly disagree

We should do more education of the public on this issue.
❑ strongly agree ❑ agree ❑ not sure ❑ disagree ❑ strongly disagree

THREE REALMS OF ETHICS*

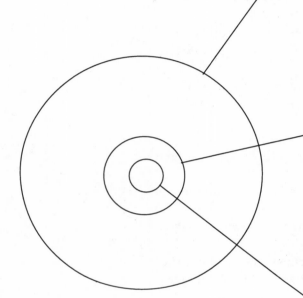

Societal The good and virtuous society
Societal Ethics deals with the common good – the overall and long-term good and goodness of a society (city, state, country). It attends to the health, vigor, balance, and equity of society's key systems and structures – political, economic, legal, educational, etc. – so that society increasingly is and continues to be an environment in which persons can be born grow, labor, love, flourish, age and die as humanely as possible. Societal ethics deals primarily with the key systems and structures of society.

Institutional The good and virtuous institution
Institutional ethics deals with the overall and long-term good and goodness of institutions (families, agencies, corporations). It attends to the health, vigor, balance, and equity of the institution's key systems and structures so that the institution can accomplish its mission while attending to its rights and duties vis-à-vis the individuals who make it up and the larger society in which it exists. Institutional ethics deals primarily with the key systems and structures of institutions.

Individual The good and virtuous individual
Individual ethics deals with the good and goodness of individuals. It attends to the balance and right relationships among various dimensions of a single individual (spiritual, mental, physical, emotional, etc.) as well as the rights and duties that exist between separate individuals. Individual ethics tends to deal with the behaviors and virtues of individuals.

*Three Realms of Ethics, John W. Glaser,
Sheed & Ward, Kansas City, MO

Center for Healthcare Ethics 440 South Batavia, Orange, CA 92668 (714) 997-7690

10 PROCESSES FOR DISCUSSING ONE ARTICLE: PROCESS 9

Purpose: To take the three-realm paradigm and examine the issue from each of these perspectives and identify key relationships between the three dimensions of the issue.

"Private and public sector leaders have an urgent civic responsibility to preserve and strengthen our nation's predominantly not-for-profit healthcare system."

Societal Issues:

1. Forces/factors on the national level that support this are....

2. Forces/factors on the national level that inhibit this are....

3. Forces/factors on the state level that support this are....

4. Forces/factors on the state level that inhibit this are....

5. Action implications for Catholic health care include.....

6. Action implications for our institution include.......

Insitutional Issues

1. This should be a clear priority for our management.
   ❑ strongly agree ❑ agree ❑ not sure ❑ disagree ❑ strongly disagree
   Comment:

2. We need to clarify and emphasize this more in our organization.
   ❑ strongly agree ❑ agree ❑ not sure ❑ disagree ❑ strongly disagree
   Comment:

3. This should find expression in the job descriptions of senior management.
   ❑ strongly agree ❑ agree ❑ not sure ❑ disagree ❑ strongly disagree
   Comment:

4. We should select board members who understand the importance of this issue.
   ❑ strongly agree ❑ agree ❑ not sure ❑ disagree ❑ strongly disagree
   Comment:

Individual Issues:

1. I personally agree with this statement.
   ❏ strongly agree ❏ agree ❏ not sure ❏ disagree ❏ strongly disagree
   Comment:

2. I have a good understanding of the nature of not-for-profit sphere of civic life and its relationship to government and business.
   ❏ strongly agree ❏ agree ❏ not sure ❏ disagree ❏ strongly disagree
   Comment:

3. I spend substantive time reflecting on and learning about this issue.
   ❏ strongly agree ❏ agree ❏ not sure ❏ disagree ❏ strongly disagree
   Comment:

4. I spend substantive time actively preserving and strengthening not-for-profit health care.
   ❏ strongly agree ❏ agree ❏ not sure ❏ disagree ❏ strongly disagree
   Comment:

5. Some things that I have done in the last six months that stand out for me in this regard are:

In light of our discussion:

- as (executive committee, as ethics committee, etc), what are some next steps that we should take?

- as (hospital, home health agency, etc.), what are some next steps that we should take?

- what systems and structures call for special attention in order to improve the situation?

10 PROCESSES FOR DISCUSSING ONE ARTICLE: PROCESS 10

Purpose: To focus on and express some of the feelings that are inevitably present but usually expressed only indirectly when discussing such issues.

(It is important to notice that there is a big difference between saying "I feel that . . ." and "I feel. . ." The former is really a way of saying what I *think* and not what I *feel*. The following exercises are intended to help us focus on our feelings and not on our thoughts.)

1. A good society needs both economic goods (cars, toasters, computers, etc.) and noneconomic goods (families, education, healthcare, etc.). It should treat these different goods in essentially different ways. *When I read this, I feel . . .*

feeling	mild	moderate	strong
harmony			
irritation			
confusion			
peace			
anger			
clarity			
frustration			
balance			
perplexity			
union			
defensiveness			
agitation			
delight			
gratitude			
loneliness			
joy			

2. There are two different kinds of social institutions: 1) those whose primary purpose is to earn a profit and reasonable rate of return on investment; 2) those whose primary purpose is to advance human dignity (family, schools, courts, cities, etc.). *When I read this, I feel . . .*

feeling	mild	moderate	strong
harmony			
irritation			
confusion			
peace			
anger			
clarity			
frustration			
balance			

feeling	mild	moderate	strong
perplexity			
union			
defensiveness			
agitation			
delight			
gratitude			
loneliness			
joy			

3. "The idea that the entirety of social life is to be determined by market exchanges is to run 'the risk of an idolatry of the market, an idolatry which ignores the existence of goods which by their nature are not and cannot be mere commodities.' " *When I read this, I feel . . .*

feeling	mild	moderate	strong
harmony			
irritation			
confusion			
peace			
anger			
clarity			
frustration			
balance			
perplexity			
union			
defensiveness			
agitation			
delight			
gratitude			
loneliness			
joy			

4. "The purpose of a not-for-profit organization is to improve the human condition, that is, to advance important noneconomic, nonregulatory functions that cannot be as well-served by either business corporations or government." *When I read this, I feel . . .*

feeling	mild	moderate	strong
harmony			
irritation			
confusion			
peace			
anger			
clarity			
frustration			
balance			
perplexity			
union			
defensiveness			
agitation			
delight			
gratitude			
loneliness			
joy			

In light of our discussion:

- as (executive committee, ethics committee, etc.), what are some next steps that we should take?

- as (hospital, home health agency, etc.), what are some next steps that we should take?

- what systems and structures call for special attention in order to improve the situation?

CHAPTER 19

28 PROCESSES FOR REFLECTION AND ACTION:

- these can be applied to articles in this book, but also to other proposals and projects of your organization;

- these are generic, highly selective, and usually include more material than can be dealt with at one meeting; so they call for tailoring to your needs;

- the more you take time to tailor these to your specific needs, the greater benefit your group will experience;

- the more an individual discussion is planned as part of a larger program of reflection, the more substantial the long-term benefits to an organization;

- no matter what the purpose of the discussion, it can always be helpful to ask at the end: given our experience during this discussion, what practical steps should we take as an organization?

1. PROCESS AS SURVEY TO SEE RANGE OF OPINIONS.

This process takes some/all key ideas from an article and asks for response/reaction. This can take various forms:

> some can be tallied and graphed to give visual feedback – some more nuanced than others: e.g., Lickert or yes/not
> > sure/no;
> some are open-ended – "what do you think about this . . ."
> some combine both: Lickert + comments.

The results of such surveys can be gathered, collated and fed back to the group before the discussion. Or the survey can simply be used to structure the discussion without any prior exposure to the article. There are a wide range of variations between these two options.

Here's one example:

1. A good society needs both economic goods (cars, toasters, computers, etc.) and noneconomic goods (families, education, healthcare, etc.). It should treat these different goods in essentially different ways.
   ❏ strongly agree ❏ agree ❏ not sure ❏ disagree ❏ strongly disagree
   Comment:

2. There are two different kinds of social institutions: 1) those whose primary purpose is to earn a profit and reasonable rate of return on investment; 2) those whose primary purpose is to advance human dignity (family, schools, courts, cities, etc.).
❏ strongly agree ❏ agree ❏ not sure ❏ disagree ❏ strongly disagree
Comment:

In light of our discussion:

- as (executive committee, ethics committee, etc.), what are some next steps that we should take?

- as (hospital, home health agency, etc.), what are some next steps that we should take?

- what systems and structures call for special attention in order to improve the situation?

2. PROCESS TO EXPLORE THE POSITIVE AND NEGATIVE ASPECTS OF STATED POSITIONS.

1. A good society needs both economic goods (cars, toasters, computers, etc.) and noneconomic goods (families, education, healthcare, etc.). It should treat these different goods in essentially different ways.

   What makes sense to me about this is:

   What does not make sense to me about this is:

2. There are two different kinds of social institutions: 1) those whose primary purpose is to earn a profit and reasonable rate of return on investment; 2) those whose primary purpose is to advance human dignity (family, schools, courts, cities, etc.).
   What makes sense to me about this is:

   What does not make sense to me about this is:

In light of our discussion:

- as (executive committee, ethics committee, etc.), what are some next steps that we should take?

- as (hospital, home health agency, etc.), what are some next steps that we should take?

- what systems and structures call for special attention in order to improve the situation?

3. A PROCESS TO EXAMINE THE SIMILARITIES AND DIFFERENCES BETWEEN MY OWN POSITION/UNDERSTANDING AND HOW I JUDGE OUR TEAM'S POSITION ON AN ISSUE.

I agree personally 1-5 5=high		Our mgt. team agrees 1-5 5=high
	1. A good society needs both economic goods (cars, toasters, computers, etc.) and noneconomic goods (families, education, healthcare, etc.). It should treat these different goods in essentially different ways.	
	2. There are two different kinds of social institutions: 1) those whose primary purpose is to earn a profit and reasonable rate of return on investment; 2) those whose primary purpose is to advance human dignity (family, schools, courts, cities, etc.).	

In light of our discussion:

- as (executive committee, ethics committee, etc.), what are some next steps that we should take?

- as (hospital, home health agency, etc.), what are some next steps that we should take?

- what systems and structures call for special attention in order to improve the situation?

4. PROCESS THAT COMPARES WHAT I THINK SHOULD BE IN OUR ORGANIZATION AND WHAT I THINK THE ACTUAL SITUATION IS.

Should be in organization		Actually is in our organization
	1. A good society needs both economic goods (cars, toasters, computers, etc.) and noneconomic goods (families, education, healthcare, etc.). It should treat these different goods in essentially different ways.	
	2. There are two different kinds of social institutions: 1) those whose primary purpose is to earn a profit and reasonable rate of return on investment; 2) those whose primary purpose is to advance human dignity (family, schools, courts, cities, etc.).	

In light of our discussion:

- as (executive committee, ethics committee, etc.), what are some next steps that we should take?

- as (hospital, home health agency, etc.), what are some next steps that we should take?

- what systems and structures call for special attention in order to improve the situation?

5. PROCESS COMPARING OUR INSTITUTION'S *RHETORIC* WITH ITS *ACTUAL BEHAVIOR.*

Our rhetoric affirms 1-5 5=high		Our behavior exhibits 1-5 5=high
	1. A good society needs both economic goods (cars, toasters, computers, etc.) and noneconomic goods (families, education, healthcare, etc.). It should treat these different goods in essentially different ways.	
	2. There are two different kinds of social institutions: 1) those whose primary purpose is to earn a profit and reasonable rate of return on investment; 2) those whose primary purpose is to advance human dignity (family, schools, courts, cities, etc.).	

In light of our discussion:

- as (executive committee, ethics committee, etc.), what are some next steps that we should take?

- as (hospital, home health agency, etc.), what are some next steps that we should take?

- what systems and structures call for special attention in order to improve the situation?

6. A PROCESS FOR COMPARING OUR ASSUMPTIONS WITH A SOLID EVIDENCE BASE FOR THESE ASSUMPTIONS.

We operate on this assumption 1-5 5=high		We have good data base for assumption 1-5 5=high
	1. A good society needs both economic goods (cars, toasters, computers, etc.) and noneconomic goods (families, education, healthcare, etc.). It should treat these different goods in essentially different ways.	
	2. There are two different kinds of social institutions: 1) those whose primary purpose is to earn a profit and reasonable rate of return on investment; 2) those whose primary purpose is to advance human dignity (family, schools, courts, cities, etc.).	

In light of our discussion:

- as (executive committee, ethics committee, etc.) what are some next steps that we should take?

- as (hospital, home health agency, etc.), what are some next steps that we should take?

- what systems and structures call for special attention in order to improve the situation?

7. A PROCESS FOR EXAMINING OUR LANGUAGE.

Our corporate language is sensitive to this 1-5		Examples of need for better expression
	1. A good society needs both economic goods (cars, toasters, computers, etc.) and noneconomic goods (families, education, healthcare, etc.). It should treat these different goods in essentially different ways.	
	2. There are two different kinds of social institutions: 1) those whose primary purpose is to earn a profit and reasonable rate of return on investment; 2) those whose primary purpose is to advance human dignity (family, schools, courts, cities, etc.).	
	3. "The idea that the entirety of social life is to be determined by market exchanges is to run 'the risk of an idolatry of the market, an idolatry which ignores the existence of goods which by their nature are not and cannot be mere commodities.'"	
	4. "The purpose of a not-for-profit organization is to improve the human condition, that is, to advance important noneconomic, nonregulatory functions that cannot be as well-served by either business corporations or government."	
	5. "The primary question in an investor-owned organization is: How do we ensure a reasonable return to our shareholders? Other questions may be asked . . . but always in the context of their effect on profit."	

In light of our discussion:

- as (executive committee, ethics committee, etc.), what are some next steps that we should take?

- as (hospital, home health agency, etc.), what are some next steps that we should take?

- what systems and structures call for special attention in order to improve the situation?

8. A PROCESS FOR ATTENDING TO FEELINGS/EMOTIONS

1. A good society needs both economic goods (cars, toasters, computers, etc.) and noneconomic goods (families, education, healthcare, etc.). It should treat these

different goods in essentially different ways. When I read this,
I feel . . .

feeling	mild	moderate	strong
harmony			
irritation			
confusion			
peace			
anger			
clarity			
frustration			
balance			
perplexity			
union			
defensiveness			
agitation			
delight			
gratitude			
loneliness			
joy			

In light of our discussion:

- as (executive committee, ethics committee, etc.), what are some next steps that we should take?

- as (hospital, home health agency, etc.), what are some next steps that we should take?

- what systems and structures call for special attention in order to improve the situation?

9. A PROCESS FOR SHARING RELIGIOUS, FAMILY, ETHNIC TRADITIONS:

1. A good society needs both economic goods (cars, toasters, computers, etc.) and noneconomic goods (families, education, healthcare, etc.). It should treat these different goods in essentially different ways.
   In my family/religious/ethnic tradition, this echoes/conflicts with . . .

2. There are two different kinds of social institutions: 1) those whose primary purpose is to earn a profit and reasonable rate of return on investment; 2) those whose primary purpose is to advance human dignity (family, schools,

courts, cities, etc.).
In my family/religious/ethnic tradition, this echoes/conflicts with . . .

3. "The idea that the entirety of social life is to be determined by market exchanges is to run 'the risk of an idolatry of the market, an idolatry which
ignores the existence of goods which by their nature are not and cannot be
mere commodities.' "
In my family/religious/ethnic tradition, this echoes/conflicts with . . .

4. "The purpose of a not-for-profit organization is to improve the human condition, that is, to advance important noneconomic, nonregulatory functions that
cannot be as well-served by either business corporations or government."
In my family/religious/ethnic tradition, this echoes/conflicts with . . .

In light of our discussion:

- as (executive committee, ethics committee, etc.), what are some next steps that
  we should take?

- as (hospital, home health agency, etc.), what are some next steps that we should
  take?

- what systems and structures call for special attention in order to improve the
  situation?

10. A PROCESS EXAMINING PERSONAL HOPES AND FEARS:

1. A good society needs both economic goods (cars, toasters, computers, etc.) and
noneconomic goods (families, education, healthcare, etc.). It should treat these
different goods in essentially different ways.
This stirs up these hopes:

This stirs up these fears:

2. There are two different kinds of social institutions: 1) those whose primary
purpose is to earn a profit and reasonable rate of return on investment; 2) those
whose primary purpose is to advance human dignity (family, schools, courts,
cities, etc.).
This stirs up these hopes:

This stirs up these fears:

3. "The idea that the entirety of social life is to be determined by market exchanges is to run 'the risk of an idolatry of the market, an idolatry which ignores the existence of goods which by their nature are not and cannot be mere commodities.'"
This stirs up these hopes:

This stirs up these fears:

4. "The purpose of a not-for-profit organization is to improve the human condition, that is, to advance important noneconomic, nonregulatory functions that cannot be as well-served by either business corporations or government."
This stirs up these hopes:

This stirs up these fears:

In light of our discussion:

- as (executive committee, ethics committee, etc.), what are some next steps that we should take?

- as (hospital, home health agency, etc.), what are some next steps that we should take?

- what systems and structures call for special attention in order to improve the situation?

11. A PROCESS FOR MAKING IMPLICIT ASSUMPTIONS EXPLICIT:

Often discussions are less productive and satisfying than we would like because the underlying assumptions at work are never raised to an explicit level and dealt with directly. This process helps to reach down and pull up our implicit assumptions so that we can identify them for ourselves and for the group.

- There is an iron law of universal access to health care: if you want universal health care coverage, then be prepared to ration; if you are not prepared to ration, abandon all hopes of an affordable plan of universal coverage.
  ❏ strongly agree ❏ agree ❏ not sure ❏ disagree ❏ strongly disagree

  Assumption(s) leading me to this position:

- Rationing should be understood as a symbol of reasoning and restraint: we can get what we need if we are prepared, in the process, to restrain ourselves.
  ❏ strongly agree ❏ agree ❏ not sure ❏ disagree ❏ strongly disagree

  Assumption(s) leading me to this position:

- "Rationing" means an action undertaken when there is: 1) a recognition that resources are limited, and b) when faced with scarcity, a method that must be devised to allocate fairly and reasonably those resources.
  ❏ strongly agree ❏ agree ❏ not sure ❏ disagree ❏ strongly disagree

  Assumption(s) leading me to this position:

- "Both because no nation on earth, not even the United States, can promise unbounded health care regardless of the cost, and because Congress will not pay for such health care, some system of limits must be put in place. I call such a system a 'rationing.' "
  ❏ strongly agree ❏ agree ❏ not sure ❏ disagree ❏ strongly disagree

  Assumption(s) leading me to this position:

- We are profoundly mistaken in believing that we should not move to open and conscious rationing *until* we have wrung all waste out of the system.
  ❏ strongly agree ❏ agree ❏ not sure ❏ disagree ❏ strongly disagree

  Assumption(s) leading me to this position:

In light of our discussion:

- as (executive committee, ethics committee, etc.), what are some next steps that we should take?

- as (hospital, home health agency, etc.), what are some next steps that we should take?

- what systems and structures call for special attention in order to improve the situation?

12. A PROCESS FOR IDENTIFYING KEY VALUES:

One way to provide consistent response to varying situations is to identify and apply key values to these variables. This exercise helps each individual identify key values related to an issue and examine these in the community of reflection.

• "The physician-patient relationship is the cornerstone for achieving, maintaining and improving health. The structure of financing and regulation should be designed to foster and support an ideal relationship between the physician and the patient."
❑ strongly agree ❑ agree ❑ not sure ❑ disagree ❑ strongly disagree

The key value on which I base my judgment is:

• "To evaluate the effects of managed care, we need to delineate an ideal conception of the physician-patient relationship."
❑ strongly agree ❑ agree ❑ not sure ❑ disagree ❑ strongly disagree

The key value on which I base my judgment is:

• "We suggest that the fundamental elements of the ideal physician-patient relationship that are embodied in our intuitions and common to ethical analyses and legal standards can be expressed as six C's: choice, competence, communication, compassion, continuity, and (no) conflict of interest."
❑ strongly agree ❑ agree ❑ not sure ❑ disagree ❑ strongly disagree

The key value on which I base my judgment is:

Some practical steps that might diminish the impediments to these elements in the physician-patient relationship include:

1) using global budgets instead of price competition among managed care plans for cost control;
❑ strongly agree ❑ agree ❑ not sure ❑ disagree ❑ strongly disagree

The key value on which I base my judgment is:

2) prohibiting all schemes that use salary incentives or bonuses tied to physician test-ordering patterns;
❑ strongly agree ❑ agree ❑ not sure ❑ disagree ❑ strongly disagree

The key value on which I base my judgment is:

3) restricting expensive advertising by managed care plans by capping their promotion budgets;
❏ strongly agree ❏ agree ❏ not sure ❏ disagree ❏ strongly disagree

The key value on which I base my judgment is:

4) requiring managed care plans to have a board of patients and physicians to approve policies regarding length of office visits and telephone calls;
❏ strongly agree ❏ agree ❏ not sure ❏ disagree ❏ strongly disagree

The key value on which I base my judgment is:

5) creating an independent review board to assess the reliability and validity of all quality indicators before they are approved or required for use by managed care plans;
❏ strongly agree ❏ agree ❏ not sure ❏ disagree ❏ strongly disagree

The key value on which I base my judgment is:

6) implementing insurance reform legislation to ensure mobility of insurance with job changes and purchasing of coverage by individuals;
❏ strongly agree ❏ agree ❏ not sure ❏ disagree ❏ strongly disagree

The key value on which I base my judgment is:

7) providing universal coverage to enable otherwise uninsured patients to have an opportunity for an ideal physician-patient relationship.
❏ strongly agree ❏ agree ❏ not sure ❏ disagree ❏ strongly disagree

The key value on which I base my judgment is:

In light of our discussion:

- as (executive committee, ethics committee, etc.), what are some next steps that we should take?

- as (hospital, home health agency, etc.), what are some next steps that we should take?

- what systems and structures call for special attention in order to improve the situation?

13. A PROCESS FOR EXAMINING THE ADVANTAGES AND DISADVANTAGES OF "RIGHTS TALK":

It is common to cast issues of health care in terms of rights. This is a powerful language for examining the ethical dimensions of managed care. But like all conceptual frameworks, "rights talk" has its strengths and weaknesses. This exercise aims at examining the pros and cons of using language of rights.

Issue from article	Reformulation in rights language	Advantages	Disadvantages
Physicians see their responsibility as loyal and uncompromised advocates of each patient's best interests as an ethical imperative at the core of medicine.	Physicians have the right . . . Or, Patients have a right . . .		
Plan members must recognize that while their physician has a responsibility to care for them, that responsibility is tempered by the duty to use the limited resources of the MCO prudently.	Physicians have a right . . . Or, Patients of MCO have a right . . . Or, MCO has a right . . .		
A physician in an MCO cannot be an *unrestricted advocate* of each patient's best interests. That is, a physician's advocacy can never ignore the needs of the rest of the MCO's members. Physicians and administrators should evaluate the MCO's advertising and be sure that it does not mislead potential plan members.			
Patients need to be educated, before joining the plan, that for the sake of cost-control they are buying an approach to health services delivery that includes limits and trade-offs.			

In light of our discussion:

- as (executive committee, ethics committee, etc.), what are some next steps that we should take?

- as (hospital, home health agency, etc.), what are some next steps that we should take?

- what systems and structures call for special attention in order to improve the situation?

14. A PROCESS FOR EXAMINING THE THREE REALMS OF AN ISSUE: SOCIETAL, INSTITUTIONAL, INDIVIDUAL

Issue	Questions/issues/ implications for us as individuals	Questions/issues implications for our organization	Questions/issues/ implications for public policy
1.			
2.			
3.			
4.			

In light of our discussion:

- as (executive committee, ethics committee, etc.), what are some next steps that we should take?

- as (hospital, home health agency, etc.), what are some next steps that we should take?

- what systems and structures call for special attention in order to improve the situation?

15. A PROCESS FOR PRESENTING POINT/COUNTERPOINT ON AN ISSUE:

Take one, two, three issues from a reading and ask two persons from your group to prepare opposing positions on these key issues. At the meeting, the opposing positions are presented to the group, with discussion following the presentations.

In light of our discussion:

- as (executive committee, ethics committee, etc.) what are some next steps that we should take?

- as (hospital, home health agency, etc.), what are some next steps that we should take?

- what systems and structures call for special attention in order to improve the situation?

16. A PROCESS FOR CONSIDERING ISSUES IN TERMS OF THEIR BURDENS AND BENEFITS:

Faced with a number of alternatives:

those alternatives are ethically good whose benefits outweigh their burdens;

those alternatives are ethically bad whose burdens outweigh their benefits;

those alternatives are ethically ambiguous where the ratio of burdens and benefits is unclear.

Explicitly examining the burdens and benefits of an issue in some detail can be an important step.

Burdens:	Issue:	Benefits:
1.		
2.		
3.		
4.		
5.		

In light of our discussion:

- as (executive committee, ethics committee, etc.), what are some next steps that we should take?

- as (hospital, home health agency, etc.), what are some next steps that we should take?

- what systems and structures call for special attention in order to improve the situation?

17. A PROCESS FOR EXAMINING THE FEASIBILITY OF AN ISSUE:

Sometimes the right thing to do is obvious but not feasible, at least at the present moment. Considering the feasibility of an issue and what needs to be done to make an obvious good a feasible goal – long/short term – is an important ethical perspective.

Issue:	Is clearly an ethical good 1-5 5=high	Degree of feasibility 1-5 5=high	Steps to make it more feasible
1.			
2.			
3.			
4.			
5.			

In light of our discussion:

- as (executive committee, ethics committee, etc.), what are some next steps that we should take?

- as (hospital, home health agency, etc.), what are some next steps that we should take?

- what systems and structures call for special attention in order to improve the situation?

18. A PROCESS FOR EXAMINING OUR ORGANIZATION – A:

This examines a broad range of organizational issues. Categories should be added, deleted, modified to fit the needs of your organization.

Issue:	We should have a consensus on this.	This is an explicit priority.	Have put this into strategic steps.	This is well-communicated through the organization.	Persons are hired in line with this.	Recognition/ rewards align with this.	Account-ability systems to track this.
1.							
2.							
3.							
4.							

In light of our discussion:

- as (executive committee, ethics committee, etc.), what are some next steps that we should take?
- as (hospital, home health agency, etc.), what are some next steps that we should take?
- what systems and structures call for special attention in order to improve the situation?

19. A PROCESS FOR EXAMINING OUR ORGANIZATION – B:

Each team member before the meeting:

- reads the article;
- picks one issue that s/he considers very important for consideration;
- fills in the response areas on the grid below (or modified grid).

At the meeting:

- each person in turn, without immediate discussion, takes the team through the issue they have identified and the responses they have made on the grid.

In light of our discussion:

- as (executive committee, ethics committee, etc.), what are some next steps that we should take?
- as (hospital, home health agency, etc.), what are some next steps that we should take?
- what systems and structures call for special attention in order to improve the situation?

20. A PROCESS FOR EXAMINING OUR ORGANIZATION – C:

Facilitator

- selects two or three issues from reading;

- sends out form (adapted to suit specific needs), which is returned to facilitator with enough time to tabulate responses before the meeting;

- tabulates and graphs responses;

- hands out collated responses at meeting to serve as basis of discussion.

Issue:	We should have a consensus on this.	This is an explicit priority.	Have put this into strategic steps.	This is well communicated through the organization.	Persons are hired in line with this.	Recognition/ rewards align with this.	Accountability systems to track this.
1.							
2.							
3.							

In light of our discussion:

- as (executive committee, ethics committee, etc.), what are some next steps that we should take?

- as (hospital, home health agency, etc.), what are some next steps that we should take?

- what systems and structures call for special attention in order to improve the situation?

21. A PROCESS FOR CLARIFYING UNDERLYING MORAL PRINCIPLES/ FUNDAMENTAL REASONS:

One way to be consistent across different value conflicts is to bring basic principles to bear on our choices. Because these principles are usually implicit and often unexamined, it can help individuals and a group to take the time to articulate and examine these principles.
❑ strongly agree ❑ agree ❑ not sure ❑ disagree ❑ strongly disagree
A key moral principle/fundamental reason that shapes my position on this is. . . .

In light of our discussion:

- as (executive committee, ethics committee, etc.), what are some next steps that we should take?

- as (hospital, home health agency, etc.), what are some next steps that we should take?

- what systems and structures call for special attention in order to improve the situation?

22. A PROCESS FOR CLARIFYING THE MEANING OF WORDS WE USE:

Not seldom the words we use are ambiguous. Each person can have a different, sometimes opposite, understanding of the words used to discuss an issue. Good ethics requires that the key concepts of a discussion be clarified and examined to uncover such divergent meanings and to develop consensual meaning.

Issue:	Key term(s) in this issue:	Term(s) mean to me:
1.		
2.		
3.		
4.		
5.		

In light of our discussion:

- as (executive committee, ethics committee, etc.), what are some next steps that we should take?

- as (hospital, home health agency, etc.), what are some next steps that we should take?

- what systems and structures call for special attention in order to improve the situation?

23. A PROCESS FOR ENHANCING ORGANIZATIONAL CONSENSUS:

Issue:	Degree of org. consensus (1-10 10=high)	Reason for my assessment	Need for change (1-10 10= high)	Levers/mechanisms important for improvement

In light of our discussion:

- as (executive committee, ethics committee, etc.), what are some next steps that we should take?

- as (hospital, home health agency, etc.), what are some next steps that we should take?

- what systems and structures call for special attention in order to improve the situation?

24. A PROCESS FOR ANALYZING THE ALLOCATION OF BURDENS/ BENEFITS IN THE DE FACTO SITUATION AND IN AN IDEAL SITUATION.

Issue:	De facto who bears/reaps major burdens/ benefits?	Examples	Ideal allocation of burdens/ benefits	Systems needing attention to improve the situation

In light of our discussion:

- as (executive committee, ethics committee, etc.), what are some next steps that we should take?

- as (hospital, home health agency, etc.), what are some next steps that we should take?

- what systems and structures call for special attention in order to improve the situation?

25. A PROCESS FOR EXAMINING MECHANISMS FOR ADDRESSING ETHICAL ISSUES IN MANAGED CARE.

Issue	Board dedicates time to understanding & addressing this problem.	Mgmt. dedicates time to understanding & addressing this problem.	Patients/staff are enabled to provide feedback.	Priorities for improvement.

In light of our discussion:

- as (executive committee, ethics committee, etc.), what are some next steps that we should take?

- as (hospital, home health agency, etc.), what are some next steps that we should take?

- what systems and structures call for special attention in order to improve the situation?

26. A PROCESS FOR IDENTIFYING MORALLY PROBLEMATIC ISSUES AND A DIRECTION FOR RESOLUTION.

Morally problematic issue	Reasons why it is morally problematic	Positive/ negative consequences of this issue	Alternative structures	Next steps

In light of our discussion:

- as (executive committee, ethics committee, etc.), what are some next steps that we should take?
- as (hospital, home health agency, etc.), what are some next steps that we should take?
- what systems and structures call for special attention in order to improve the situation?

27. A PROCESS FOR EXAMINING SYSTEMS OF COMMUNICATION.

Issue:	How important to share this information (1-10 10= high)?	How effective in sharing with staff?	How effective in sharing with patients?	Priorities for improvement

In light of our discussion:

- as (executive committee, ethics committee, etc.), what are some next steps that we should take?
- as (hospital, home health agency, etc.), what are some next steps that we should take?
- what systems and structures call for special attention in order to improve the situation?

28. A PROCESS FOR EXAMINING COLLABORATION.

Issue	Collaboration across departments? De facto/ideal?	Collaboration with community agencies?	De facto/ideal? Collaboration with religious congregations? De facto/ideal?

In light of our discussion:

- as (executive committee, ethics committee, etc.), what are some next steps that we should take?

- as (hospital, home health agency, etc.), what are some next steps that we should take?

- what systems and structures call for special attention in order to improve the situation?

FOR FURTHER READING

Biblo, Joan D., and Myra J. Christopher, Linda Johnson, and Robert Lyman Potter, *Ethical Issues in Managed Care: Guidelines for Clinicians and Recommendations to Accrediting Organizations.* Kansas City, MO: Midwest Bioethics Group, 1995.

Chapman, Audrey, ed., *Health Care Reform: A Human Rights Approach.* Washington, D.C.: Georgetown University Press, 1994.

Churchill, Larry, *Rationing Health Care in America: Perceptions and Principles of Justice.* Notre Dame, IN: University of Notre Dame Press, 1987.

Dougherty, John, *Back to Reform: Values, Markets, and the Health Care System.* New York: Oxford University Press, 1996.

Eddy, David, *Clinical Decision Making,* London, Jones and Bartlett Publishers, 1996.

Glaser, John, *Three Realms of Ethics.* Kansas City, MO: Sheed & Ward, 1994.

Keane, Philip, *Health Care Reform: A Catholic View.* New York: Paulist Press, 1993.

LaPuma, John and David Schiedermayer, *Pocket Guide to Managed Care: Business, Practice, Laws, and Ethics.* New York: McGraw Hill, 1996.

Morreim, E. Haavi, *Balancing Act: The New Medical Ethics of Medicine's New Economics.* Washington, D.C.: Georgetown University Press, 1995.

National Health Council, *Putting Patients First.* Washington, D.C.: National Health Council, 1996.

Priester, Reinhard, *Taking Values Seriously: A Values Framework for the U.S. Health Care System.* Minneapolis, MN: The Center for Biomedical Ethics, 1992.

Rodwin, Marc A., *Medicine, Money, and Morals: Physicians' Conflicts of Interests.* New York: Oxford University Press, 1993.

Thurston, Jeffrey M., *Death of Compassion: The Endangered Doctor-Patient Relationship.* Waco, TX: WRS Publishing, 1996.

Woodstock Theological Center, *Ethical Considerations in the Business Aspects of Health Care.* Washington, D.C.: Georgetown University Press, 1995.